Medical Pharmacology
at a Glance

Medical Pharmacology at a Glance

MICHAEL J. NEAL
Professor and Chairman of the
Division of Pharmacology and Toxicology
United Medical and Dental Schools
of Guy's and St Thomas's Hospitals (UMDS)
Department of Pharmacology
St Thomas's Hospital, London

THIRD EDITION

**Blackwell
Science**

© 1987, 1992, 1997 by
Blackwell Science Ltd
Editorial Offices:
Osney Mead, Oxford OX2 0EL
25 John Street, London WC1N 2BS
23 Ainslie Place, Edinburgh EH3 6AJ
350 Main Street, Malden
    MA 02148 5018, USA
54 University Street, Carlton
    Victoria 3053, Australia
10, rue Casimir Delavigne
    75006 Paris, France

Other Editorial Offices:
Blackwell Wissenschafts-Verlag GmbH
Kurfürstendamm 57
10707 Berlin, Germany

Blackwell Science KK
MG Kodenmacho Building
7–10 Kodenmacho Nihombashi
Chuo-ku, Tokyo 104, Japan

Iowa State University Press
A Blackwell Science Company
2121 S. State Avenue
Ames, Iowa 50014-8300, USA

Printed and bound in Great Britain by
MPG Books Ltd, Bodmin, Cornwall

First published 1987
Reprinted 1988, 1989 (twice), 1990, 1991 (twice)
Four Dragons edition 1989
Reprinted 1991
Second edition 1992
Reprinted 1993 (twice), 1994, 1995 (twice), 1996
Four Dragons edition 1992
Reprinted 1993 (twice), 1994, 1995
Third edition 1997
Reprinted 1997, 1998, 2000, 2001

A catalogue record for this title
is available from the British Library

ISBN 0-86542-719-4 (BSL)
ISBN 0-632-04816-6 (IE)

Library of Congress
Cataloging-in-Publication Data

Neal, M.J.
    Medical pharmacology at a glance/
    Michael J. Neal—3rd ed.
        p.   cm.
    Includes bibliographical references and index.
    ISBN 0-86542-719-4
    1 Pharmacology.   I. Title.
    [DNLM: 1 Pharmacology, Clinical.
    QV 38 N342m 1997]
    RM300.N38 1997
    615'.1—dc21
    DNLM/DLC   97–2123
    for Library of Congress   CIP

DISTRIBUTORS

Marston Book Services Ltd
PO Box 269
Abingdon
Oxon OX14 4YN
(*Orders:* Tel: 01235 465500
            Fax: 01235 465555)

USA
    Blackwell Science, Inc.
    Commerce Place
    350 Main Street
    Malden, MA 02148 5018
    (*Orders:* Tel: 800 759 6102
                      781 388 8250
               Fax: 781 388 8255)

Canada
    Login Brothers Book Company
    324 Saulteaux Crescent
    Winnipeg, Manitoba R3J 3T2
    (*Orders:* Tel: 204 837 2987)

Australia
    Blackwell Science Pty Ltd
    54 University Street
    Carlton, Victoria 3053
    (*Orders:* Tel: 03 9347-0300
               Fax: 03 9347-5001)

For further information on
Blackwell Science, visit our website:
www.blackwell-science.com

Contents

Preface

This book is written primarily for medical students but it should also be useful to students and scientists in other disciplines who would like an elementary and concise introduction to pharmacology.

In this book the text has been reduced to a minimum for understanding the figures. Nevertheless, I have attempted in each chapter to explain how the drugs produce their effects and to outline their uses.

In this third edition most chapters have been updated and new chapters have been added on lipid-lowering drugs, antiemetics, anthelmintics, poisoning and adverse drug reactions.

Acknowledgements

I am grateful to Professor J. Ritter and Dr E. Joyce who kindly read chapters relating to their special interest and who offered valuable advice and criticism. I am especially grateful to Miss Jean Plaskett for preparing the manuscript, and to the many students who have written appreciative letters and who have made helpful suggestions.

How to use this book

Each of the chapters (listed on p. 5) represents a particular topic, corresponding roughly to a 60-minute lecture. Beginners in pharmacology should start at Chapter 1 and first read through the text on the left-hand pages (which occasionally continues to the facing right-hand page above the ruled line) of several chapters using the figures only as a guide.

Once the general outline has been grasped, it is probably better to concentrate on the *figures* one at a time. Some are quite complicated and can certainly not be taken in 'at a glance'. Each should be studied carefully and worked through together with the *legends* (right-hand pages). Since many drugs appear in more than one chapter, considerable cross-referencing has been provided. As progress is made through the book, use of this cross-referencing will provide valuable reinforcement and a greater understanding of drug action. Once the information has been understood, the figures should subsequently require little more than a brief look to refresh the memory.

The figures are highly diagrammatic and not to scale.

Further reading

British National Formulary. British Medical Association and The Royal Pharmaceutical Society of Great Britain, London (about 700 pp). The BNF is updated twice a year.

Rang, H.P. & Dale, M.M. (1995) *Pharmacology*, 3rd edn. Churchill Livingstone, Edinburgh (855 pp).

Ritter, J.M., Lewis, L.D. & Mant, G.K. (1995) *Textbook of Clinical Pharmacology*, 3rd edn. Edward Arnold, London (725 pp).

1 Introduction: principles of drug action

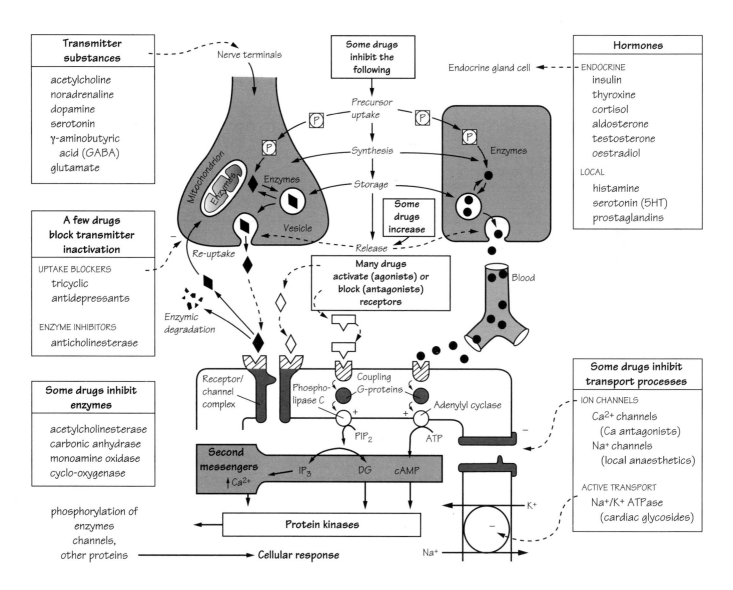

Medical pharmacology is the science of chemicals (drugs) that interact with the human body. These interactions are divided into two classes:
- **pharmacodynamics**, the effects of the drug on the body, and
- **pharmacokinetics**, the way the body affects the drug with time (i.e. absorption, distribution, metabolism and excretion).

The most common ways in which a drug can produce its effects are shown in the figure. A few drugs (e.g. general anaesthetics, osmotic diuretics) act by virtue of their physicochemical properties and this is called **non-specific** drug action. Some drugs act as false substrates or inhibitors for certain **transport systems** (bottom right) or **enzymes** (bottom left). Most drugs, however, produce their effects by acting on specific protein molecules, usually located in the cell membrane. These proteins are called **receptors** ( ) and they normally respond to endogenous chemicals in the body. These chemicals are either synaptic **transmitter substances** (top left, ◆) or **hormones** (top right, ●). For example, acetylcholine is a transmitter substance released from motor nerve endings and it activates receptors in skeletal muscle, initiating a sequence of events that results in contraction of the muscle. Chemicals (e.g. acetylcholine) or drugs that activate receptors and produce a response are called **agonists**. Some drugs, called **antagonists** ( ), combine with receptors, but do not activate them. Antagonists reduce the probability of the transmitter substance (or another agonist) combining with the receptor and so reduce or block its action.

The activation of receptors by an agonist or hormone is coupled to the physiological or biochemical responses by transduction mechanisms (lower figure) that often (but not always) involve molecules called '**second messengers**' ( ).

The interaction between a drug and the binding site of the receptor depends on the complementarity of 'fit' of the two molecules. The closer the fit and the greater the number of bonds (usually non-covalent), the stronger will be the attractive forces between them, and the higher the **affinity** of the drug for the receptor. The ability of a drug to combine with one particular type of receptor is called **specificity**. No drug is truly specific but many have a relatively **selective** action on one type of receptor.

Drugs are prescribed to produce a therapeutic effect but they often produce additional **unwanted effects** (Chapter 45) that range from the trivial (e.g. slight nausea) to the fatal (e.g. aplastic anaemia).

RECEPTORS

These are protein molecules which are normally activated by transmitters or hormones. Many receptors have now been cloned and their amino acid sequences determined. The four main types of receptor are listed below.

1 Agonist (ligand) gated channels made up of protein subunits which form a central pore (e.g. nicotinic receptor, Chapter 6; γ-aminobutyric acid (GABA) receptor, Chapter 24).

2 G-protein coupled receptors (see below) form a family of receptors with seven membrane-spanning helices. They are linked to physiological responses by second messengers.

3 Receptors for steroid hormones (Chapter 34) and thyroid hormones (Chapter 35) are present on the cell nucleus and regulate transcription and thus protein synthesis.

4 Insulin receptors are directly linked to tyrosine kinase (Chapter 36).

Transmitter substances are chemicals released from nerve terminals and which diffuse across the synaptic cleft and bind to the receptors. This activates the receptors, presumably by changing their conformation, and triggers a sequence of post-synaptic events resulting in, for example, muscle contraction or glandular secretion. Following its release, the transmitter is inactivated (left of figure) by either enzymic degradation (e.g. acetylcholine) or reuptake (e.g. noradrenaline, GABA). Many drugs act by either reducing or enhancing synaptic transmission.

Hormones are chemicals released into the bloodstream; they produce their physiological effects on tissues possessing the necessary specific hormone receptors. Drugs may interact with the endocrine system by inhibiting (e.g. antithyroid drugs, Chapter 35) or increasing (e.g. oral antidiabetic agents, Chapter 36) hormone release. Other drugs interact with hormone receptors which may be activated (e.g. steroidal anti-inflammatory drugs, Chapter 33) or blocked (e.g. oestrogen antagonists, Chapter 34). Local hormones (autacoids) such as histamine, serotonin (5-hydroxytryptamine, 5HT), kinins and prostaglandins are released in pathological processes. The effects of histamine can sometimes be blocked with antihistamines (Chapter 11), and drugs that block prostaglandin synthesis (e.g. aspirin) are widely used as anti-inflammatory agents (Chapter 32).

TRANSPORT SYSTEMS

The lipid cell membrane provides a barrier against the transport of hydrophilic molecules into or out of the cell.

Ion channels are selective pores in the membrane that allow the ready transfer of ions down their electrochemical gradient. The open–closed state of these channels is controlled either by the membrane potential (voltage-gated channels) or by transmitter substances (ligand-gated channels). Some channels (e.g. Ca^{2+} channels in the heart) are both voltage and transmitter gated. Voltage-gated channels for sodium, potassium and calcium have the same basic structure (Chapter 5) and subtypes exist for each different channel. Important examples of drugs that act on voltage-gated channels are *calcium antagonists* (Chapter 16) that block L-type calcium channels in vascular smooth muscle and the heart, and *local anaesthetics* (Chapter 5) that block sodium channels in

nerves. Some *anticonvulsants* (Chapter 25) and some *anti-arrhythmic* drugs (Chapter 17) also block Na^+ channels. No clinically useful drug acts primarily on voltage-gated K^+ channels but *oral antidiabetic* drugs act on a different type of K^+ channel that is regulated by intracellular adenosine triphosphate (ATP; Chapter 36).

Active transport processes are used to transfer substances against their concentration gradients. They utilize special carrier molecules in the membrane and require metabolic energy. Two examples are listed below.

1 *Sodium pump*. This expels Na^+ ions from inside the cell by a mechanism that derives energy from ATP and involves the enzyme adenosine triphosphatase (ATPase). The carrier is linked to the transfer of K^+ ions into the cell. The *cardiac glycosides* (Chapter 18) act by inhibiting the Na^+/K^+ ATPase. Na^+ and/or Cl^- transport processes in the kidney are inhibited by some *diuretics* (Chapter 14).

2 *Noradrenaline transport*. The *tricyclic antidepressants* (Chapter 28) prolong the action of noradrenaline by blocking its reuptake into central nerve terminals.

ENZYMES

These are catalytic proteins that increase the *rate* of chemical reactions in the body. Drugs that act by inhibiting enzymes include: *anticholinesterases*, which enhance the action of acetylcholine (Chapters 6 and 8); *carbonic anhydrase inhibitors*, which are diuretics (i.e. increase urine flow, Chapter 14); *monoamine oxidase inhibitors*, which are antidepressants (Chapter 28); and inhibitors of *cyclo-oxygenase* (e.g. aspirin, Chapter 32).

SECOND MESSENGERS

These are chemicals whose intracellular concentration increases or, more rarely, decreases in response to receptor activation by agonists, and which trigger processes that eventually result in a cellular response. The most studied second messengers are: Ca^{2+} ions, cyclic adenosine monophosphate (cAMP), inositol-1,4,5-trisphosphate ($InsP_3$) and diacylglycerol (DG).

cAMP is formed from ATP by the enzyme adenylyl cyclase when, for example, β-adrenoceptors are stimulated. The cAMP activates an enzyme (protein kinase A) which phosphorylates a protein (enzyme or ion channel) and leads to a physiological effect.

$InsP_3$ and DG are formed from membrane phosphatidylinositol 4,5-bisphosphate by activation of a phospholipase C. Both messengers can, like cAMP, activate kinases, but $InsP_3$ does this indirectly by mobilizing intracellular calcium stores. Some muscarinic effects of acetylcholine and $α_1$-adrenergic effects involve this mechanism (Chapter 7).

G-proteins. The stimulation of adenylyl cyclase and phosphokinase C following receptor activation is mediated by a family of regulatory guanosine triphosphate (GTP)-binding proteins (G-proteins). The receptor–agonist complex induces a conformational change in the G-protein, causing its α-subunit to bind GTP. α-GTP dissociates from the G-protein and activates (or inhibits) the enzyme. The signal to the enzyme ends because α-GTP has intrinsic GTPase activity and turns itself off by hydrolysing the GTP to GDP. α-GDP then reassociates with the βγ G-protein subunits.

9

2 Drug–receptor interactions

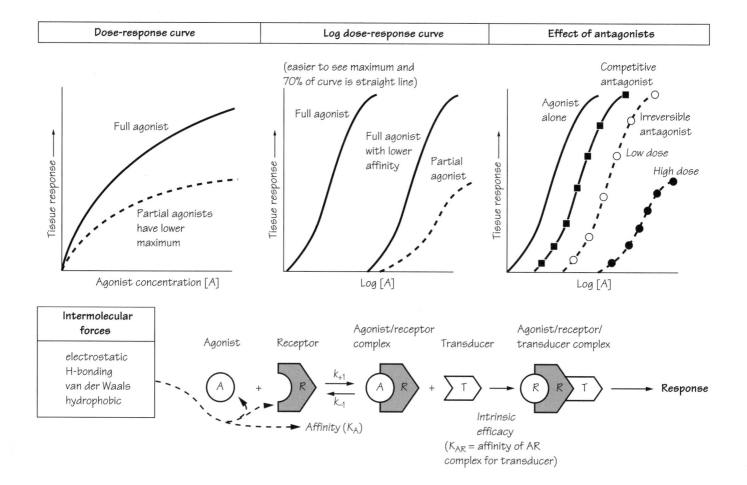

Dose-response curve	Log dose-response curve	Effect of antagonists

The tissues in the body have only a few basic responses when exposed to agonists (e.g. muscle contraction, glandular secretion) and the quantitative relationship between these physiological responses and the concentration of the agonist can be measured by using **bioassays**. The first part of the drug–receptor interaction, i.e. the binding of drug to receptor, can be studied in isolation using **binding assays**.

It has been found by experiment that for many tissues and agonists, when the response is plotted against the concentration of the drug, a curve is produced that is often hyperbolic (**dose–response curve**, top left). In practice, it is often more convenient to plot the response against the logarithm of the agonist concentration (**log dose–response curve**, middle top). Assuming the interaction between the drug (A) and the receptor (R) (lower figure) obeys the law of mass action, then the concentration of drug–receptor complex (AR) is given by:

$$[AR] = \frac{[R_O][A]}{K_D + [A]}$$

where R_O = total concentration of receptors, A = agonist concentration, K_D = dissociation constant, and AR = concentration of occupied receptors.

Since this is the equation for a hyperbola, the shape of the dose–response curve is explained if the response is directly proportional to [AR]. Unfortunately, this simple theory does not explain another experimental finding—some agonists, called **partial agonists**, cannot elicit the same maximum response as full agonists even if they have the same affinity for the receptor (top left and middle, - - -). Thus, in addition to having affinity for the receptor, an agonist has another chemical property called **intrinsic efficacy**, which is its ability to elicit a response when it binds to a receptor (lower figure).

A **competitive antagonist** has no intrinsic efficacy and effectively dilutes the receptor concentration. This causes a parallel shift of the log dose–response curve to the right (top right,■) but the maximum response is not depressed. In contrast, **irreversible antagonists** depress the maximum response (top right,●). However, at low concentrations a parallel shift of the log dose–response curve may occur without a reduction in the maximum response (top right, ○). Since an irreversible antagonist in effect removes receptors from the system, it is clear that not all the receptors need to be occupied to elicit the maximum response (i.e. there is a receptor reserve).

INTERMOLECULAR FORCES

Drug molecules in the environment of receptors are attracted initially by relatively long-range electrostatic forces. Then, if the molecule is suitably shaped to fit closely to the binding site of the receptor, hydrogen bonds and van der Waals forces briefly bind the drug to the receptor. Irreversible antagonists bind to receptors with strong covalent bonds.

AFFINITY

This is a measure of how avidly a drug binds to its receptor. It is characterized by the equilibrium dissociation constant (K_D), which is the ratio of rate constants for the reverse (k_{-1}) and forward (k_{+1}) reaction between the drug and the receptor. The reciprocal of K_D is called the affinity constant (K_A) and (in the absence of receptor reserve, see below) is the concentration of drug that produces 50% of the maximum response.

ANTAGONISTS

These are drugs that bind to receptors but do not activate them. They may be competitive or irreversible.

Competitive antagonists bind reversibly with receptors and the tissue response can be returned to normal by increasing the dose of agonist, because this increases the probability of agonist–receptor collisions at the expense of antagonist–receptor collisions. The ability of higher doses of agonist to overcome the effects of the antagonist results in parallel shift of the dose–response curve to the right and is the hallmark of competitive antagonism.

Irreversible antagonists (e.g. phenoxybenzamine) have an effect which cannot be reversed by increasing the concentration of agonist.

RECEPTOR RESERVE

In many tissues, irreversible antagonists initially shift the log dose–response curve to the right without reducing the maximum response, indicating that the maximum response can be obtained without the agonist occupying all the receptors. The excess receptors are sometimes called '*spare*' receptors, but this is a misleading term because they are of functional significance. They increase both the sensitivity and speed of a system because the concentration of drug–receptor complex (and hence the response) depends on the product of the agonist concentration and the *total* receptor concentration.

PARTIAL AGONIST

This is an agonist that cannot elicit the same maximum response as a 'full' agonist. The reasons for this are unknown. Recently, it has been suggested that agonism depends on the affinity of the drug–receptor complex for a *transducer molecule* (lower figure). Thus, a full agonist produces a complex with high affinity for the transducer (e.g. the coupling G-proteins, Chapter 1), whilst a partial agonist–receptor complex has a lower affinity for the transducer and so cannot elicit the full response.

When acting at receptors alone, partial agonists stimulate a physiological response, but they antagonize the effects of a full agonist (e.g. some β-adrenoceptor antagonists, Chapters 15 and 16).

INTRINSIC EFFICACY

This is the ability of an agonist to alter the conformation of a receptor in such a way that it elicits a response in the system. It is defined as the affinity of the agonist–receptor complex for a transducer.

Partial agonists and receptor reserve. A drug that is a partial agonist in a tissue with no receptor reserve may be a full agonist in a tissue possessing many 'spare' receptors, because its poor efficacy can be offset by activating a larger number of receptors than that required by a full agonist.

BIOASSAY

Bioassays involve the use of a biological tissue to relate drug concentration to a physiological response. Usually, isolated tissues are used because it is then easier to control the drug concentration around the tissue and reflex responses are abolished. Bioassays can be used to estimate:

- the concentration of a drug;
- its binding constants; or
- its potency relative to another drug.

Measurement of the relative potencies of a series of agonists on different tissues has been one of the main ways used to classify receptors, e.g. adrenoceptors (Chapter 7).

BINDING ASSAYS

Binding assays are simple and very adaptable. Membrane fragments from homogenized tissues are incubated with radiolabelled drug (usually ^3H) and then recovered by filtration. After correction for non-specific binding, the ^3H-drug bound to the receptors can be determined and estimations made of K_A and B_{max} (number of binding sites). Binding assays are widely used to study drug receptors but have the disadvantage that no functional response is measured, and often the radiolabelled drug does not bind to a single class of receptor.

3 Drug absorption, distribution and excretion

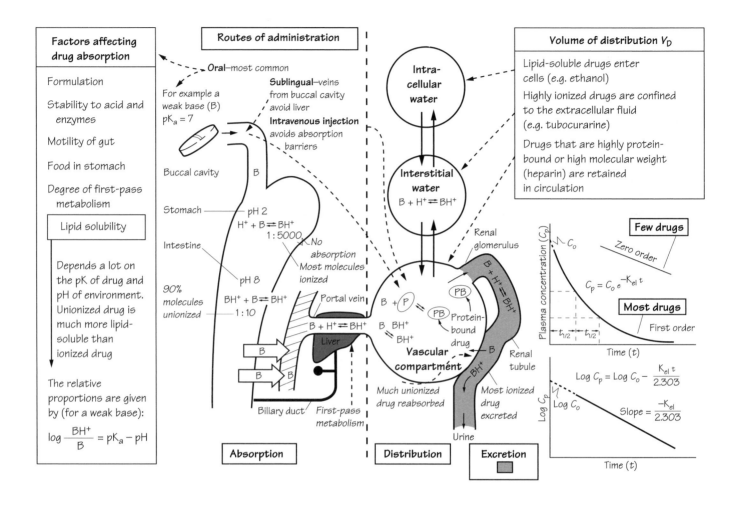

Most drugs are given **orally** and they must pass through the gut wall to enter the bloodstream (left of figure, ⇨). This **absorption** process is affected by many factors (left) but is usually proportional to the **lipid solubility** of the drug. Thus, the absorption of unionized molecules (B) is favoured because they are far more lipid soluble than those that are ionized (BH$^+$) and surrounded by a 'shell' of water molecules. Drugs are absorbed mainly from the small intestine because of its large surface area. This is true even for weak acids (e.g. aspirin) which are non-ionized in the acid (HCl) of the stomach. Drugs absorbed from the gastrointestinal tract enter the portal circulation (left, ▨) and some are extensively metabolized as they pass through the liver (first-pass metabolism).

Drugs that are sufficiently lipid soluble to be readily absorbed orally are rapidly distributed throughout the body water compartments (◯). Many drugs are loosely bound to plasma albumin, and an equilibrium forms between the bound (PB) and free (B) drug in the plasma. Drug that is bound to plasma proteins is confined to the vascular system and is not able to exert its pharmacological actions.

If a drug is given by **intravenous injection**, it enters the blood and is rapidly distributed to the tissues. By taking repeated blood samples, the fall in plasma concentration of the drug with time (i.e. the rate of drug elimination) can be measured (right, top graph). Often the concentration falls rapidly at first, but then the rate of decline progressively decreases. Such a curve is called **exponential**, and this means that at any given time a **constant fraction** of the drug present is eliminated in unit time. Many drugs show an exponential fall in plasma concentration because the rates at which the drug elimination processes work are themselves usually proportional to the concentration of drug in the plasma. The following processes are involved.

1 Elimination in the urine by glomerular filtration (right, ▨).
2 Metabolism, usually by the liver.
3 Uptake by the liver and subsequent elimination in the bile (solid line from liver).

A process that depends on the concentration at any given time is called **first order** and most drugs exhibit first-order elimination kinetics. If any enzyme system responsible for drug metabolism becomes **saturated**, then the elimination kinetics change to **zero order**, i.e. the rate of elimination proceeds at a constant rate and is unaffected by an increased concentration of the drug (e.g. ethanol, phenytoin).

ROUTES OF ADMINISTRATION

Drugs can be administered orally or parenterally (i.e. by a non-gastrointestinal route).

Oral. Most drugs are absorbed by this route and because of its convenience it is the most widely used. However, some drugs (e.g. benzylpenicillin, insulin) are destroyed by the acid or enzymes in the gut and must be given parenterally.

Intravenous injection enters the drug directly into the circulation and bypasses the absorption barriers. It is used:
- where a rapid effect is required (e.g. frusemide in pulmonary oedema);
- for continuous administration (infusion);
- for large volumes; and
- for drugs that cause local tissue damage if given by other routes (e.g. cytotoxic drugs).

Intramuscular and subcutaneous injections. Drugs in aqueous solution are usually absorbed fairly rapidly, but absorption can be slowed by giving the drug in the form of an ester (e.g. neuroleptic depot preparations; see Chapter 27).

Other routes include *inhalation* (e.g. volatile anaesthetics, some drugs used in asthma), and *topical* (e.g. ointments). *Sublingual* and *rectal* administration avoid the portal circulation, and sublingual preparations in particular are valuable in administering drugs subject to a high degree of first-pass metabolism.

DISTRIBUTION AND EXCRETION

Distribution around the body occurs when the drug reaches the circulation. It must then penetrate tissues to act.

$t_{1/2;}$ (half-life) is the time taken for the concentration of drug in blood to fall by half its original value (right, top graph). Measurement of $t_{1/2;}$ allows calculation of the *elimination rate constant* (K_{el}) from the formula:

$$K_{el} = \frac{0.69}{t}$$

K_{el} is the fraction of drug present at any time that would be eliminated in unit time (e.g. $K_{el} = 0.02$ minute^{-1} means that 2% of the drug present is eliminated in 1 minute).

The exponential curve of plasma concentration (C_p) against time (t) is described by:

$$C_p = C_0 \, e^{-K_{el}t}$$

where C_0 = the initial apparent plasma concentration. By taking logarithms, the exponential curve can be transformed into a more convenient straight line (right, bottom graph) from which C_0 and $t_{1/2}$ can readily be determined.

Volume of distribution (V_D). This is the apparent volume into which the drug is distributed. Following an intravenous injection,

$$V_D = \frac{\text{dose}}{C_0}$$

A value of $V_D < 5$ litres implies that the drug is retained within the vascular compartment. A value < 15 litres suggests that the drug is restricted to the extracellular fluid, whilst large volumes of distribution ($V_D > 15$ litres) indicate distribution throughout the total body water or concentration in certain tissues. The volume of distribution can be used to calculate the *clearance* of the drug.

Clearance is an important concept in pharmacokinetics. It is the volume of blood or plasma cleared of drug in unit time. Plasma clearance (Cl_p) is given by the relationship:

$$Cl_p = V_D K_{el}$$

The rate of elimination = $Cl_p \times C_p$. Clearance is the sum of individual clearance values. Thus, $Cl_p = Cl_m$ (metabolic clearance) + Cl_r (renal excretion). Clearance, but not $t_{1/2;}$ provides an indication of the ability of the liver and kidney to dispose of drugs.

Drug dosage. Clearance values can be used to plan dosage regimens. Ideally in drug treatment, a steady-state plasma concentration ($C_{p\,ss}$) is required within a known therapeutic range. A steady state will be achieved when the rate of drug entering the systemic circulation (dosage rate) equals the rate of elimination. Thus, the dosing rate = $Cl \times C_{p\,ss}$. This equation could be applied to an intravenous infusion because all the dose enters the circulation at a known rate. For oral administration, the equation becomes:

$$\frac{\text{F} \times \text{dose}}{\text{dosing interval}} = Cl_p \times C_p, \text{ average}$$

where F = *bioavailability* of the drug. The $t_{1/2;}$ value of a drug is useful in choosing a dosing interval that does not produce excessively high peaks (toxic levels) and low troughs (ineffective levels) in drug concentration.

Bioavailability is a term used to describe the proportion of administered drug reaching the systemic circulation. Bioavailability is 100% following an intravenous injection ($F = 1$), but drugs are usually given orally and the proportion of the dose reaching the systemic circulation varies with different drugs and also from patient to patient. Drugs subject to a high degree of first-pass metabolism may be almost inactive orally (e.g. glyceryl trinitrate, lignocaine).

EXCRETION

Renal excretion is ultimately responsible for the elimination of most drugs. Drugs appear in the glomerular filtrate, but if they are lipid soluble they are readily reabsorbed in the renal tubules by passive diffusion. Metabolism of a drug often results in a less lipid-soluble compound, aiding renal excretion (see Chapter 4).

The ionization of weak acids and bases depends on the pH of the tubular fluid. Manipulation of the urine pH is sometimes useful in increasing renal excretion. For example, bicarbonate administration makes the urine alkaline; this ionizes aspirin, making it less lipid soluble and increasing its rate of excretion.

Weak acids and weak bases are actively secreted in the proximal tubule. Penicillins are eliminated by this route.

Biliary excretion. Some drugs (e.g. stilboestrol) are concentrated in the bile and excreted into the intestine where they may be reabsorbed. This enterohepatic circulation increases the persistence of a drug in the body.

4 Drug metabolism

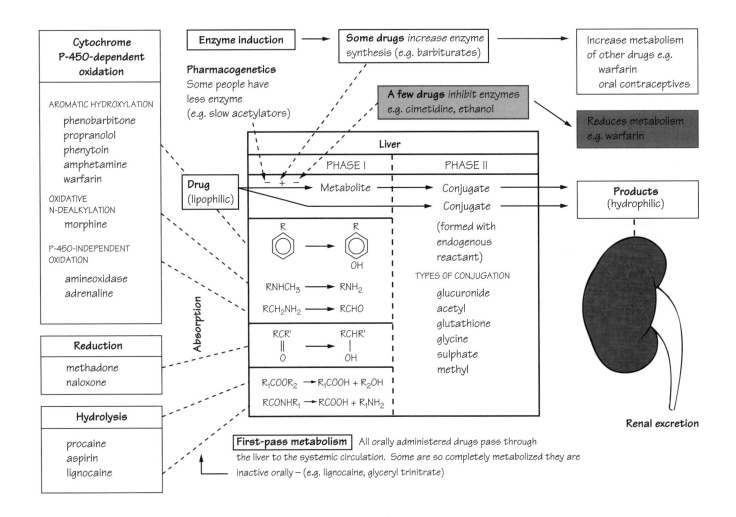

Drug metabolism has two important effects:

1 The drug is made more **hydrophilic**—this hastens its excretion by the kidneys (right, ▨) because the less lipid-soluble metabolite is not readily reabsorbed in the renal tubules.

2 The metabolites are usually **less active** than the parent drug. However, this is not always so, and sometimes the metabolites are as active as (or more active than) the original drug. For example, diazepam (a drug used to treat anxiety) is metabolized to nordiazepam and oxazepam, both of which are active. **Prodrugs** are inactive until they are metabolized in the body to the active drug. For example, levodopa, an anti-Parkinsonian drug (Chapter 26), is metabolized to dopamine, whilst the hypotensive drug methyldopa (Chapter 15) is metabolized to α-methylnoradrenaline.

The **liver** is the main organ of drug metabolism and is involved in two general types of reaction.

Phase I reactions involve the biotransformation of a drug to a more polar metabolite (left of figure) by introducing or unmasking a functional group (e.g. –OH, –NH$_2$, –SH).

Oxidations are the most common reactions and these are catalysed by an important class of enzymes called the mixed function oxidases (**cytochrome P-450s**). The substrate specificity of this enzyme complex is very low and many different drugs can be oxidized (examples, top left). Other phase I reactions are **reductions** (middle left) and **hydrolysis** (bottom left).

Phase II reactions. Drugs or phase I metabolites that are not sufficiently polar to be excreted rapidly by the kidneys are made more hydrophilic by **conjugation** with endogenous compounds in the liver (centre of figure).

Repeated administration of some drugs (top) increases the synthesis of cytochrome P-450 (**enzyme induction**). This increases the rate of metabolism of the inducing drug and also of other drugs metabolized by the same enzyme (top right). In contrast, drugs sometimes **inhibit** microsomal enzyme activity (top, ▨) and this increases the action of drugs metabolized by the same enzyme (top right, ▨).

In addition to these drug–drug interactions, the metabolism of drugs may be influenced by **genetic factors** (pharmacogenetics), age and some diseases, especially those affecting the liver.

DRUGS

A few drugs (e.g. gallamine, Chapter 6) are highly polar because they are fully ionized at physiological pH values. Such drugs are metabolized little, if at all, and the termination of their actions depends mainly on renal excretion. Most drugs, however, are highly lipophilic and are often bound to plasma proteins. Since the protein-bound drug is not filtered at the renal glomerulus and the free drug readily diffuses back from the tubule into the blood, such drugs would have a very prolonged action if their removal relied on renal excretion alone. In general, drugs are metabolized to more polar compounds, which are more easily excreted by the kidneys.

LIVER

The main organ of drug metabolism is the liver, but other organs, such as the gastrointestinal tract and lungs, have considerable activity. Drugs given orally are usually absorbed in the small intestine and enter the portal system to the liver, where they may be extensively metabolized (e.g. lignocaine, morphine, propranolol). This is called *first-pass metabolism*, a term that does not refer only to hepatic metabolism. For example, chlorpromazine is metabolized more in the intestine than by the liver.

PHASE I REACTIONS

The most common reaction is *oxidation*. Other, relatively uncommon, reactions are *reduction* and *hydrolysis*.

Microsomal mixed function oxidase system. Many of the enzymes involved in drug metabolism are located on the smooth endoplasmic reticulum, which forms small vesicles when the tissue is homogenized. These vesicles can be isolated by differential centrifugation and are called microsomes.

Microsomal drug oxidations involve nicotinamide-adenine-dinucleotide phosphate (reduced form) (NADPH), oxygen and two key enzymes: (i) a flavoprotein, NADPH-cytochrome P-450 reductase; and (ii) a haemoprotein, cytochrome P-450, which acts as a terminal oxidase. Cytochrome P-450 exists in a large number of subtypes (isoenzymes) with different, but often overlapping, substrate specificities.

PHASE II REACTIONS

These usually occur in the liver and involve conjugation of a drug or its phase I metabolite with an endogenous substance. The resulting conjugates are almost always less active and are polar molecules that are readily excreted by the kidneys.

FACTORS AFFECTING DRUG METABOLISM

Enzyme induction. Some drugs (e.g. *phenobarbitone, carbamazepine, ethanol and, especially, rifampicin*) and pollutants (e.g. *polycyclic aromatic hydrocarbons* in tobacco smoke) increase the activity of drug-metabolizing enzymes. The mechanisms involved are unclear but the chemicals somehow affect specific DNA sequences 'switching-on' the production of the appropriate enzyme, which is usually a cytochrome P-450 subtype(s). However, not all enzymes subject to induction are microsomal. For example, hepatic alcohol dehydrogenase occurs in the cytoplasm.

Enzyme inhibition may cause adverse drug interactions. They tend to occur more rapidly than those involving enzyme induction because they occur as soon as the inhibiting drug reaches a high enough concentration to compete with the affected drug. Drugs may inhibit different forms of cytochrome P-450 and so affect the metabolism only of drugs metabolized by that particular isoenzyme. *Cimetidine* inhibits the metabolism of several potentially toxic drugs including phenytoin, warfarin and theophylline. Erythromycin also inhibits the cytochrome P-450 system and increases the activity of theophylline, warfarin, carbamazepine and digoxin.

Genetic polymorphisms. The study of how genetic determinants affect drug action is called *pharmacogenetics*. The response to drugs varies between individuals and because the variations usually have a Gaussian distribution, it is assumed that the determinant of the response is multifactorial. However, some drug responses show discontinuous variation and in these cases the population can be divided into two or more groups, suggesting a single-gene polymorphism. An important example of polymorphism is *debrisoquine hydroxylation*. About 8% of the population are poor hydroxylators and show exaggerated and prolonged responses to drugs such as propranolol and metoprolol (Chapter 15), which undergo extensive hepatic metabolism.

Drug-acetylating enzymes. Hepatic *N*-acetylase displays genetic polymorphism. About 50% of the population acetylate isoniazid (an antitubercular drug) rapidly, whilst the other 50% acetylate it slowly. Slow acetylation is due to an autosomal recessive gene that is associated with decreased hepatic *N*-acetylase activity. Slow acetylators are more likely to accumulate the drug and to experience adverse reactions. There is evidence for polymorphism in the acetylation of other drugs (e.g. hydralazine, procainamide).

Plasma pseudocholinesterase. Four separate genes for this enzyme occur at one locus. Rarely ($<1:2500$), an atypical form of the enzyme occurs and this extends the duration of action of suxamethonium (a frequently used neuromuscular blocking drug) from about 6 minutes to over 2 hours or more.

Age. Hepatic microsomal enzymes and renal mechanisms are reduced at birth, especially in preterm babies. Both systems develop rapidly during the first four weeks of life. There are various methods for calculating paediatric doses (see *British National Formulary*).

In the elderly, hepatic metabolism of drugs may be reduced but declining renal function is usually more important. By 65 years, the glomerular filtration rate (GFR) decreases by 30%, and every following year it falls a further 1–2% (due to cell loss and decreased renal blood flow). Thus, older people need smaller doses of many drugs than does a younger person, especially centrally acting drugs (e.g. opioids, benzodiazepines, antidepressants), to which the elderly seem to become more sensitive (by unknown changes in the brain).

METABOLISM AND DRUG TOXICITY

Occasionally, reactive products of drug metabolism are toxic to various organs, especially the liver. *Paracetamol*, a widely used weak analgesic, normally undergoes glucuronidation and sulphation. However, these processes become saturated at high doses and the drug is then conjugated with glutathione. If the glutathione supply becomes depleted, then a reactive and potentially lethal hepatotoxic metabolite accumulates (Chapter 44).

5 Local anaesthetics

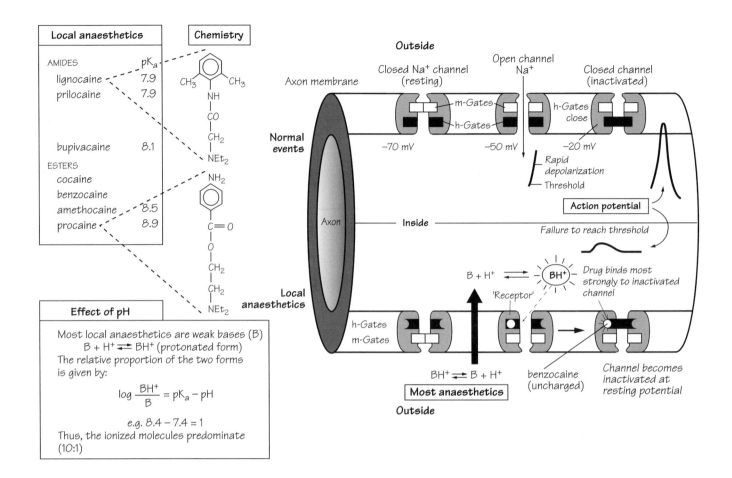

Local anaesthetics (top left) are drugs used to prevent pain by causing a reversible block of conduction along nerve fibres. Most are weak bases that exist mainly in a protonated form at body pH (bottom left). The drugs penetrate the nerve in a non-ionized (lipophilic) form (➡), but once inside the axon, some ionized molecules are formed and these block the Na⁺ channels, (▣) preventing the generation of **action potentials** (lower figure).

All nerve fibres are sensitive to local anaesthetics but, in general, small-diameter fibres are more sensitive than large fibres. Thus, a **differential block** can be achieved where the smaller pain and autonomic fibres are blocked, whilst coarse touch and movement fibres are spared. Local anaesthetics vary widely in their potency, duration of action, toxicity and ability to penetrate mucous membranes.

Local anaesthetics depress other excitable tissues (e.g. myocardium) if the concentration in the blood is sufficiently high, but their main systemic effects involve the central nervous system. Synthetic agents produce sedation and light-headedness, although anxiety and restlessness sometimes occur, presumably because central inhibitory synapses are depressed. Higher, toxic doses cause twitching and visual disturbances, whilst severe toxicity causes convulsions and coma, with respiratory and cardiac depression, resulting from medullary depression. Even cocaine, which has central stimulant properties unrelated to its local anaesthetic action, may cause death by respiratory depression.

Lignocaine is the most widely used agent. It acts more rapidly and is more stable than most other local anaesthetics. It has a duration of action of about 90 minutes. **Prilocaine** is similar to lignocaine but is more extensively metabolized and is less toxic in equipotent doses. **Bupivacaine** has a slow onset (up to 30 minutes) but a very long duration of action, up to 8 hours when used for nerve blocks. It is often used in pregnancy to produce continuous epidural blockade during labour. **Benzocaine** is a neutral, water-insoluble, local anaesthetic of low potency. Its only use is in **surface anaesthesia** for non-inflamed tissue (e.g. mouth and pharynx). The more toxic agents, **amethocaine** and **cocaine**, have restricted use. Cocaine is primarily used for surface anaesthesia where its intrinsic vasoconstrictor action is desirable (e.g. in the nose). Amethocaine drops are used in ophthalmology to anaesthetize the cornea, but less toxic drugs such as **oxybuprocaine** and **proxymetacaine**, which cause much less initial stinging, are better.

Hypersensitivity reactions may occur with local anaesthetics, especially in atopic patients, and more often with procaine and other esters of *p*-aminobenzoic acid.

Na⁺ CHANNELS

Excitable tissues possess special voltage-gated Na^+ channels that consist of one large glycoprotein α-subunit and sometimes two smaller β-subunits of unknown function. The α-subunit has four identical domains, each containing six membrane-spanning α-helices (S1–S6). The 24 cylindrical helices are stacked together radially in the membrane to form a central channel. Exactly how voltage-gated channels work is not known, but their conductance (gNa^+) is given by $gNa^+ = \bar{g}Na^+ \, m^3h$, where $\bar{g}Na^+$ is the maximum conductance possible, and m and h are gating constants that depend on the membrane potential. In the figure, these constants are shown schematically as physical gates within the channel. At the resting potential, most h-gates are open and the m-gates are closed (closed channel). Depolarization causes the m-gates to open (open channel) but the intense depolarization of the action potential then causes the h-gates to close the channel (inactivation). This sequence is shown in the upper half of the figure (left to right). The m-gate may correspond to the four positively charged S4 helices, which are thought to open the channel by moving outwards and rotating in response to membrane depolarization. The h-gate responsible for inactivation may be the intracellular loop connecting the S3 and S5 helices; this swings into the internal mouth of the channel.

ACTION POTENTIAL

If enough Na^+ channels are opened, then the rate of Na^+ entry into the axon exceeds the rate of K^+ exit and at this point, the threshold potential, entry of Na^+ ions further depolarizes the membrane. This opens more Na^+ channels, resulting in further depolarization which opens more Na^+ channels and so on. The fast inward Na^+ current quickly depolarizes the membrane towards the Na^+ equilibrium potential (around +67 mV). Then, inactivation of the Na^+ channels and the continuing efflux of K^+ ions causes repolarization of the membrane. Finally, the Na^+ channels regain their normal 'excitable' state and the Na^+ pump restores the lost K^+ and removes the gained Na^+ ions.

MECHANISM OF LOCAL ANAESTHETICS

Local anaesthetics *penetrate* into the interior of the axon in the form of the lipid-soluble free base. There, protonated molecules are formed which then enter and *block* the Na^+ channels after binding to a '*receptor*'. Thus, quaternary (fully protonated) local anaesthetics work only if they are injected inside the nerve axon. Uncharged agents (e.g. benzocaine) dissolve in the membrane but the channels are blocked in an all-or-none manner. Thus, ionized and non-ionized molecules act in essentially the same way; that is, by binding to a 'receptor' on the Na^+ channel. This 'blocks' the channel, largely by preventing the opening of h-gates (i.e. by increasing inactivation). Eventually, so many channels are inactivated that their number falls below the minimum necessary for depolarization to reach threshold, and because action potentials cannot be generated, nerve block occurs. Local anaesthetics are 'use dependent'; that is, the degree of block is proportional to the rate of nerve stimulation. This indicates that more drug molecules (in their protonated form) enter the Na^+ channels when they are open and cause more inactivation.

CHEMISTRY

Commonly used local anaesthetics consist of a lipophilic end (often an aromatic ring) and a hydrophilic end (usually a secondary or tertiary amine), connected by an intermediate chain that incorporates an ester or amide linkage.

EFFECTS

These may be:
1 *local* and include nerve blockade and direct effects on vascular smooth muscle;
2 *regional*, comprising loss of sensations (pain, temperature, touch) and vasomotor tone in the region supplied by the blocked nerves; and
3 *systemic* effects, occurring because of absorption or intravenous administration.

Heart. The effects of local anaesthetics on the *heart* are discussed in Chapter 17. Cardiac toxicity probably does not occur in subconvulsive doses.

Vascular smooth muscle. The local effects vary. **Cocaine** is a vasoconstrictor (because it blocks noradrenaline reuptake and potentiates sympathetic activity), whilst **procaine** is a vasodilator. Most *amides* cause vasoconstriction at low concentrations and vasodilatation at higher concentrations. **Prilocaine** is most likely to produce vasoconstriction at clinical doses, followed by **lignocaine** and **bupivacaine**. The regional effect is vasodilatation caused by blockade of sympathetic nerves.

Duration of action. In general, high potency and long duration are related to high lipid solubility because this results in much of the locally applied drug entering the cells. Vasoconstriction also tends to prolong the anaesthetic effect by reducing systemic distribution of the agent, and this can be achieved by the addition of a vasoconstrictor such as adrenaline, noradrenaline or felypressin (a peptide). Vasoconstrictors must not be used for producing ring-block of an extremity (e.g. finger or toe) because they may cause prolonged ischaemia and gangrene.

Amides are dealkylated in the liver and esters (not cocaine) are hydrolysed by plasma pseudocholinesterase, but drug metabolism has little effect on the duration of action of agents actually in the tissues.

METHODS OF ADMINISTRATION

Surface anaesthesia. Topical application to external or mucosal surfaces.

Infiltration anaesthesia. Subcutaneous injection to act on local nerve endings, usually with a vasoconstrictor.

Nerve block. Techniques range from infiltration of anaesthetic around a single nerve (e.g. dental anaesthesia) to epidural and spinal anaesthesia. In spinal anaesthesia (intrathecal block) a drug is injected into the cerebrospinal fluid in the subarachnoid space. In epidural anaesthesia, the anaesthetic is injected outside the dura. Spinal anaesthesia is technically far easier to produce than epidural anaesthesia, but the latter technique virtually eliminates the post-anaesthetic complications such as headache.

Intravenous regional anaesthesia. Anaesthetic is injected intravenously into an exsanguinated limb. A tourniquet prevents the agent reaching the systemic circulation.

6 Drugs acting at the neuromuscular junction

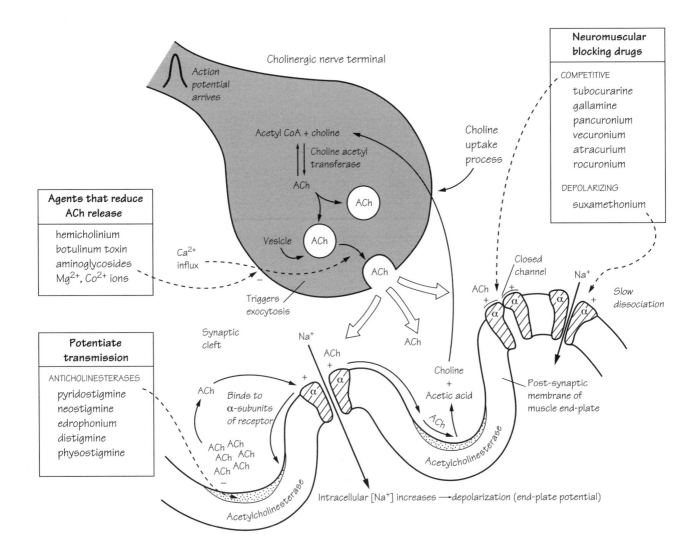

Action potentials are conducted along the motor nerves to their terminals (upper figure, ▨) where the depolarization initiates an influx of Ca^{2+} ions and the release of **acetylcholine** (ACh) by a process of **exocytosis** (⇨). The acetylcholine diffuses across the junctional cleft and binds to **receptors** located on the surface of the muscle-fibre membrane at the motor end-plate. The reversible combination of acetylcholine and receptors (lower figure, ▨) triggers the opening of cation-selective channels in the end-plate membrane, allowing an influx of Na^+ ions and a lesser efflux of K^+ ions. The resulting depolarization, which is called an end-plate potential (EPP), depolarizes the adjacent muscle-fibre membrane. If large enough, this depolarization results in an action potential and muscle contraction. The acetylcholine released into the synaptic cleft is rapidly hydrolysed by an enzyme, acetylcholinesterase (▦), which is present in the end-plate membrane close to the receptors.

Neuromuscular transmission can be increased by **anticholinesterase drugs** (bottom left) which inhibit acetylcholinesterase and slow down the hydrolysis of acetylcholine in the synaptic cleft (see also Chapter 8). *Neostigmine* and *pyridostigmine* are used in the treatment of **myasthenia gravis** and to reverse competitive neuromuscular

blockade after surgery. Overdosage of anticholinesterases results in excess acetylcholine and a depolarization block of motor end-plates (cholinergic weakness). The muscarinic effects of acetylcholine (see Chapter 7) are also potentiated by anticholinesterases but are blocked with atropine.

Neuromuscular blocking drugs (right) are used by anaesthetists to relax skeletal muscles during surgical operations and to prevent muscle contractions during electroconvulsive therapy (ECT). Most of the clinically useful neuromuscular blocking drugs compete with acetylcholine for the receptor but do not initiate ion channel opening. These 'competitive' drugs reduce the end-plate depolarizations produced by acetylcholine to a size which is below the threshold for muscle action potential generation and so cause a flaccid paralysis. **Depolarizing blockers** also act on acetylcholine receptors, but trigger the opening of the ion channels. They are not reversed by anticholinesterases. **Suxamethonium** is the only drug of this type used clinically.

Some agents (top left) act presynaptically and block neuromuscular transmission by preventing the release of acetylcholine.

Acetylcholine is synthesized in motorneurone terminals from choline and acetylcoenzyme-A by the enzyme choline acetyltransferase. The choline is taken up into the nerve endings from the extracellular fluid by a special choline carrier located in the terminal membrane.

Exocytosis. Acetylcholine is stored in nerve terminals in the cytoplasm and within synaptic vesicles (each vesicle containing about 1000–3000 acetylcholine molecules). When an action potential invades the terminal, Ca^{2+} ions enter and cause the vesicles to collide with the outer terminal membrane. This results in the release of a few hundred 'packets' or 'quanta' of acetylcholine in about a millisecond. This is called quantal release and is very sensitive to the extracellular Ca^{2+} ion concentration. Divalent ions, such as Mg^{2+}, Co^{2+} and Mn^{2+}, antagonize Ca^{2+} influx and inhibit transmitter release.

Acetylcholine receptor. This can be activated by nicotine and for this reason is called a **nicotinic receptor.** * The receptor–channel complex is constructed from four different protein subunits (denoted β, γ, δ and 2 αs) that span the membrane and are arranged to form a central pore (channel) through which cations (mainly Na^+) flow. Acetylcholine molecules bind to the two α-subunits inducing a conformational change that opens the channel for about 1 millisecond.

Myasthenia gravis is an autoimmune disease in which neuromuscular transmission is defective. Circulating heterogeneous immunoglobulin G (IgG) antibodies cause a loss of functional acetylcholine receptors in skeletal muscle. To counteract the loss of, or damage to, receptors, the amount of acetylcholine in the synaptic cleft is increased by the administration of an anticholinesterase. Immunological treatment includes administration of prednisolone or azathioprine (Chapter 43). Plasmaphoresis, in which blood is removed and the cells returned, may improve motor function, presumably by reducing the level of immune complexes. Thymectomy may be curative.

PRESYNAPTIC AGENTS

Drugs inhibiting acetylcholine release. Botulinum toxin is produced by *Clostridium botulinum* (an anaerobic bacillus, see Chapter 37). The exotoxin is extraordinarily potent and prevents acetylcholine release by an unknown mechanism. *C. botulinum* is very rarely responsible for serious food poisoning in which the victims exhibit progressive parasympathetic and motor paralysis. **Botulinium toxin type A** is used in the treatment of certain dystonias, such as blepharospasm (spasmodic eye closure) and strabismus (squint). In these conditions, low doses of toxin are injected into the appropriate muscle to produce paralysis that persists for about 12 weeks.

Aminoglycoside antibiotics (e.g. gentamicin) may cause neuromuscular blockade by inhibiting the calcium influx required for exocytosis. This unwanted effect usually occurs only as the result of an interaction with neuromuscular blockers. Myasthenia gravis may be exacerbated.

COMPETITIVE NEUROMUSCULAR BLOCKING DRUGS

In general, the competitive neuromuscular blocking drugs are bulky, rigid molecules and most have two quaternary N atoms. Neuromuscular blocking drugs are given by intravenous injection and are distributed in the extracellular fluid. They do not pass the blood–brain barrier or the placenta. The choice of a particular drug is often determined by the side effects produced. These include histamine release, vagal blockade, ganglion blockade and sympathomimetic actions. The onset of action and the duration of action of neuromuscular blocking drugs depends on the dose, but also on other factors (e.g. prior use of suxamethonium, anaesthetic agent used — enflurane in particular has a potentiating action).

Tubocurarine was introduced in 1942 and has a relatively long duration of action (30–60 minutes). It blocks ganglia, causing hypotension. Tubocurarine causes histamine release in some patients and this may lower the blood pressure further.

Gallamine does not block ganglia or release histamine but causes undesirable tachycardia by blocking the M_2-muscarinic receptors, the subtype of acetylcholine receptor that predominates in the heart (Chapter 7).

Pancuronium is a steroidal neuromuscular blocking drug with a relatively long duration of action. It does not block ganglia or cause histamine release. However, it has a dose-related atropine-like effect on the heart that produces tachycardia.

Vecuronium and atracurium are the most used agents. Vecuronium has no cardiovascular effects. It depends on hepatic inactivation and recovery can occur within 20–30 minutes, making it an attractive drug for short procedures. Atracurium has a duration of action of 15–30 minutes. It is only stable when kept cold and at low pH. At body pH and temperature it decomposes spontaneously in plasma and therefore does not depend on renal or hepatic function for its elimination. It is the drug of choice in patients with severe renal or hepatic disease. Atracurium may cause histamine release with flushing and hypotension.

Rocuronium is a new drug with a duration of action of about 30 minutes but with rapid onset of action (1–2 minutes) comparable to that of suxamethonium (1–1.5 minutes). It is reported to have no cardiovascular effects.

DEPOLARIZING NEUROMUSCULAR BLOCKING DRUGS

Suxamethonium (succinylcholine) is used because of its rapid onset and very short duration of action (3–7 minutes). The drug is normally hydrolysed rapidly by plasma pseudocholinesterase, but a few people inherit an atypical form of the enzyme and in such individuals the neuromuscular block may last for hours. Suxamethonium depolarizes the end-plate and because the drug does not dissociate rapidly from the receptors, a prolonged receptor activation is produced. The resulting end-plate depolarization initially causes a brief train of muscle action potentials and muscle-fibre twitches. Neuromuscular block then occurs as a result of several factors which include: (i) inactivation of the voltage-sensitive Na^+ channels in the surrounding muscle-fibre membrane, so that action potentials are no longer generated; and (ii) transformation of the activated receptors to a 'desensitized' state, unresponsive to acetylcholine. The main disadvantage of suxamethonium is that the initial asynchronous muscle-fibre twitches cause damage which often results in muscle pains the next day. The damage also causes potassium release. Repeated doses of suxamethonium may cause bradycardia in the absence of atropine (a muscarinic effect).

---

*Pentameric nicotinic receptors also occur in autonomic ganglia and the brain. They have variants of the α- and β-subunit and a different pharmacology.

7 Autonomic nervous system

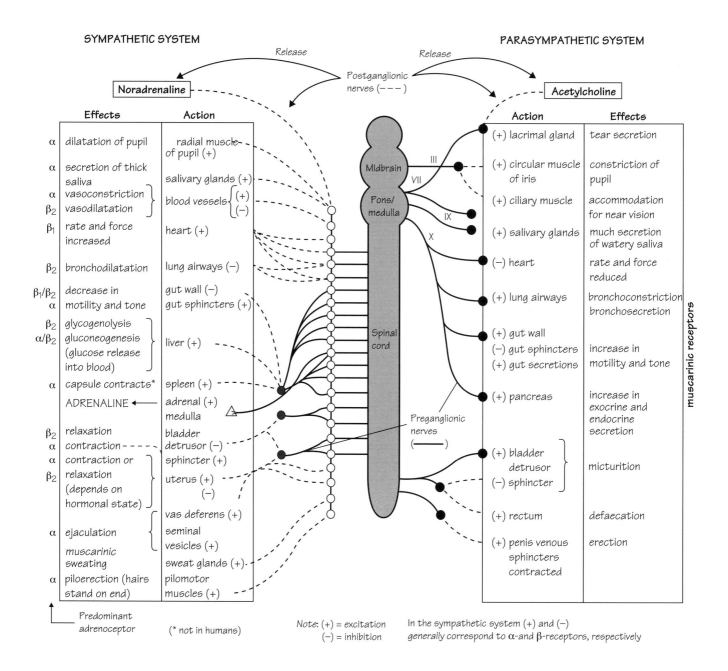

Many systems of the body (e.g. digestion, circulation) are controlled automatically by the autonomic nervous system (and the endocrine system). Control of the autonomic nervous system often involves negative feedback and there are many afferent (sensory) fibres which carry information to centres in the hypothalamus and medulla. These centres control the outflow of the autonomic nervous system, which is divided on anatomical grounds into two major parts: the **sympathetic system** (left) and the **parasympathetic system** (right). Many organs are innervated by both systems, which in general have opposing actions. The actions of sympathetic (left) and parasympathetic (right) stimulation on different tissues are indicated in the inner columns and the resulting effects on different organs are shown in the outer columns.

The sympathetic nerves (left, ——) leave the thoracolumbar region

of the spinal cord (T1–L3) and synapse either in the **paravertebral ganglia** ○ or in the **prevertebral ganglia** ● and plexuses in the abdominal cavity. Postganglionic non-myelinated nerve fibres (left, - - - -) arising from neurones in the ganglia innervate most organs of the body (left).

The transmitter substance released at sympathetic nerve endings is **noradrenaline** (top left). Inactivation of this transmitter occurs largely by reuptake into the nerve terminals. Some preganglionic sympathetic fibres pass directly to the adrenal medulla △ which can release adrenaline into the circulation. Noradrenaline and adrenaline produce their actions on effector organs by acting on α-, β_1- or β_2-**adrenoceptors** (extreme left).

In the parasympathetic system, the preganglionic fibres (right, ——)

leave the central nervous system via the cranial nerves (especially III, VII, IX and X) and the third and fourth sacral spinal roots. They often travel much further than sympathetic fibres before synapsing in ganglia (●) which are often in the tissue itself (right).

The nerve endings of the postganglionic parasympathetic fibres (right, - - - -) release **acetylcholine** (top right), which produces its actions on the effector organs (right) by activating muscarinic recep-

tors. Acetylcholine released at synapses is inactivated by the enzyme acetylcholinesterase.

All the preganglionic nerve fibres (sympathetic and parasympathetic, ——) are myelinated and release acetylcholine from the nerve terminals; the acetylcholine depolarizes the ganglionic neurones by activating nicotinic receptors.

Adrenaline mimics most sympathetic effects, i.e. it is a *sympathomimetic agent* (Chapter 9). Elliot suggested in 1904 that adrenaline was the sympathetic transmitter substance, but Dale pointed out in 1910 that *noradrenaline* mimicked sympathetic nerve stimulation more closely.

Effects of sympathetic stimulation. These are most easily remembered by thinking of what changes in the body are appropriate in the '*fright or flight reaction*'. Note which of the following effects are excitatory and which are inhibitory.
1 Pupillary dilatation (more light reaches the retina).
2 Bronchiolar dilatation (facilitates increased ventilation).
3 Heart rate and force are increased; blood pressure rises (more blood for increased activity of skeletal muscles—running!).
4 Vasoconstriction in skin and viscera and vasodilatation in skeletal muscles (appropriate redistribution of blood to muscles).
5 To provide extra energy, glycogenolysis is stimulated and the blood glucose level increases. The gastrointestinal tract and urinary bladder relax.

Adrenoceptors are divided into two main types: α-*receptors* mediate the excitatory effects of sympathomimetic amines, whilst their inhibitory effects are generally mediated by β-*receptors* (exceptions are the smooth muscle of the gut, where α-stimulation is inhibitory, and the heart, where β-stimulation is excitatory). Responses mediated by α-receptors and β-receptors can be distinguished by: (i) phentolamine and propranolol, which *selectively* block α- and β-receptors respectively; and (ii) by the relative potencies, on different tissues, of noradrenaline (NA), adrenaline (A) and isoprenaline (I). The order of potency is $NA > A > I$ where excitatory (α) responses are examined, but for inhibitory (β) responses this order is reversed (i.e. $I >> A > NA$).

β-Adrenoceptors are not homogeneous. For example, noradrenaline is an effective stimulant of cardiac β-receptors, but has little or no action on the β-receptors mediating vasodilatation. On the basis of the type of differential sensitivity they exhibit to drugs, β-receptors are divided into two types: β_1 (heart, intestinal smooth muscle) and β_2 (bronchial, vascular and uterine smooth muscle).

α-Adrenoceptors have been divided into two classes, originally depending on whether their location was postsynaptic (α_1) or presynaptic (α_2). Stimulation of the presynaptic α_2-receptors by synaptically released noradrenaline reduces further transmitter release (negative feedback). Postsynaptic α_2-receptors occur in a few tissues, e.g. brain, vascular smooth muscle (but mainly α_1).

Acetylcholine is the transmitter substance released by the following.
1 All preganglionic autonomic nerves (i.e. both sympathetic and parasympathetic).

2 All postganglionic parasympathetic nerves.
3 Some postganglionic sympathetic nerves (i.e. thermoregulatory sweat glands and skeletal muscle vasodilator fibres).
4 Nerve to adrenal medulla.
5 Somatic motor nerves to skeletal muscle end-plates (Chapter 6).
6 Some neurones in the central nervous system (Chapter 22).

Acetylcholine receptors (cholinoceptors) are divided into nicotinic and muscarinic subtypes (originally determined by measuring the sensitivity of various tissues to the drugs nicotine and muscarine, respectively).

Muscarinic receptors. Acetylcholine released at the nerve terminals of postganglionic parasympathetic fibres acts on muscarinic receptors and can be blocked selectively by atropine. Three subtypes of muscarinic receptor exist: M_1, M_2 and M_3. M_1-receptors occur in the brain and gastric parietal cells, M_2-receptors in the heart and M_3-receptors in smooth muscle and glands. Except for **pirenzepine**, which selectively blocks M_1-receptors (Chapter 12), clinically useful muscarinic agonists and antagonists show little or no selectivity for the different subtypes of muscarinic receptor.

Nicotinic receptors occur in autonomic ganglia and in the adrenal medulla, where the effects of acetylcholine (or nicotine) can be blocked selectively with hexamethonium. The nicotinic receptors at the skeletal muscle neuromuscular junction are not blocked by hexamethonium, but are blocked by tubocurarine. Thus, receptors at ganglia and neuromuscular junctions are different, although both types are stimulated by nicotine and therefore called nicotinic.

ACTIONS OF ACETYLCHOLINE

Muscarinic effects are mainly parasympathomimetic (except sweating and vasodilatation), and in general are the opposite to those caused by sympathetic stimulation. Muscarinic effects include: constriction of the pupil, accommodation for near vision (Chapter 10), profuse watery salivation, bronchiolar constriction, bronchosecretion, hypotension (due to bradycardia and vasodilatation), an increase in gastrointestinal motility and secretion, contraction of the urinary bladder and sweating.

Nicotinic effects include stimulation of all autonomic ganglia. However, the action of acetylcholine on ganglia is relatively weak compared with its effect on muscarinic receptors and so parasympathetic effects predominate. The nicotinic actions of acetylcholine on the sympathetic system can be demonstrated, for example, on cat blood pressure, by blocking its muscarinic actions with atropine. High intravenous doses of acetylcholine then cause a rise in blood pressure, because stimulation of the sympathetic ganglia and adrenal medulla now results in vasoconstriction and tachycardia.

8 Autonomic drugs acting at cholinergic synapses

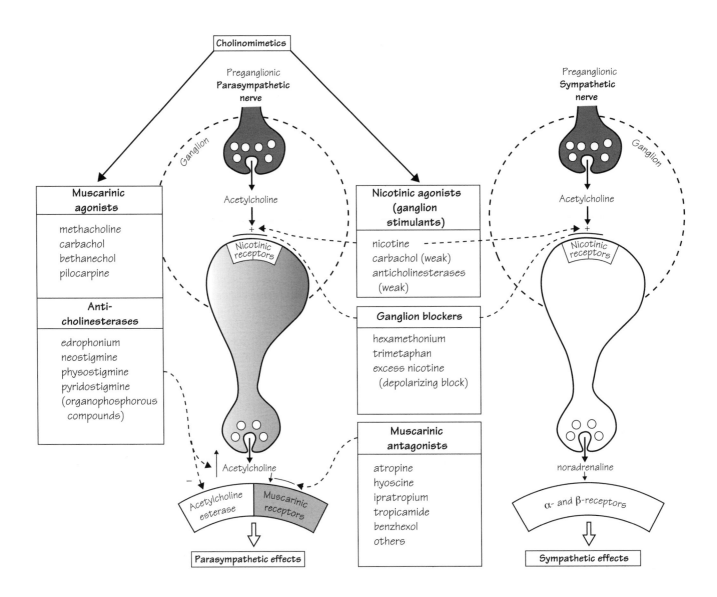

Acetylcholine released from the terminals of postganglionic parasympathetic nerves (left, ▨) produces its actions on various effector organs by activating **muscarinic receptors** (▨). The effects of acetylcholine are usually excitatory, but an important exception is the heart, which receives inhibitory cholinergic fibres from the vagus (Chapter 17). Drugs which mimic the effects of acetylcholine are called **cholinomimetics** and can be divided into two groups:
• drugs that act directly on receptors (**nicotinic and muscarinic agonists**); and
• **anticholinesterases**, which inhibit acetylcholinesterase, and so act indirectly by allowing acetylcholine to accumulate in the synapse and produce its effects.

Muscarinic agonists (top left) have few uses, but **pilocarpine** (as eyedrops) is used to reduce intraocular pressure in patients with glaucoma (Chapter 10). **Carbachol** or **bethanechol** are very occasionally used to stimulate the gut in postoperative ileus and the bladder in urinary retention under conditions where there is no obstruction to the bladder outlet (e.g. in neurological disease or postoperatively).

Anticholinesterases (bottom left) have relatively little effect at ganglia and are used mainly for their nicotinic effects on the neuromuscular junction. They are used in the treatment of myasthenia gravis and to reverse the effects of competitive muscle relaxants used during surgery (Chapter 6).

Muscarinic antagonists (bottom middle) block the effects of acetylcholine released from postganglionic parasympathetic nerve terminals. Their effects can, in general, be worked out by examination of the figure in Chapter 7. However, parasympathetic effector organs vary in their sensitivity to the blocking effect of antagonists. Secretions of the salivary, bronchial and sweat glands are most sensitive to blockade. Higher doses of antagonist dilate the pupils, paralyse accommodation and produce tachycardia by blocking vagal tone in the heart. Still higher doses inhibit parasympathetic control of the gastrointestinal tract and bladder. Gastric acid secretion is most resistant to blockade (Chapter 12).

Atropine, hyoscine (scopolamine) or other antagonists are used:
1 in anaesthesia to block vagal slowing of the heart and to inhibit

bronchial secretion;

2 to reduce intestinal spasm in, for example, irritable bowel syndrome;

3 to reduce gastric acid secretion (pirenzepine, Chapter 12);

4 in Parkinsonism (benzhexol, Chapter 26);

5 to prevent motion sickness (hyoscine, Chapter 30);

6 to dilate the pupil for ophthalmological examination (e.g. tropi-camide) or to paralyse the ciliary muscle (Chapter 10); and

7 as a bronchodilator in asthma (ipratropium, Chapter 11).

Transmission at autonomic ganglia ( ) can be stimulated by nicotinic agonists (top middle) or blocked by drugs that act specifically on the ganglionic neurone nicotinic receptor/ionophore (middle). Nicotinic agonists are of no clinical use but ganglion blockers have a limited use in anaesthesia.

Cholinergic nerve terminals in the autonomic nervous system synthesize, store and release acetylcholine in essentially the same way as at the neuromuscular junction (Chapter 6). Acetylcholinesterase is bound to both the pre- and postsynaptic membranes.

CHOLINOMIMETICS

Ganglion stimulants. These have widespread actions because they stimulate nicotinic receptors on both parasympathetic and sympathetic ganglionic neurones. Sympathetic effects include vasoconstriction, tachycardia and hypertension. Parasympathetic effects include increased motility of the gut and increased salivary and bronchial secretion. They have no clinical uses.

Muscarinic agonists. These directly activate muscarinic receptors usually producing excitatory effects. An important exception is the heart, where activation of the predominantly M_2-receptors has inhibitory effects on the rate and force of (atrial) contraction. The M_2-receptors are negatively coupled by a G-protein (G_I) to adenylyl cyclase which explains the negative inotropic effect of ACh. Subunits ($\beta\gamma$) of G_I directly increase K conductances in the heart causing hyperpolarization and bradycardia (Chapter 17). ACh stimulates glandular secretion and causes contraction of smooth muscle by activating M_3-receptors which are coupled to the formation of $InsP_3$ and diacylglycerol (Chapter 1). $InsP_3$ increases cytosolic Ca^{2+}, thus triggering muscle contraction or glandular secretion. An intravenous injection of ACh causes vasodilatation indirectly by releasing nitric oxide (NO) from vascular endothelial cells (Chapter 16). However, most blood vessels have no parasympathetic innervation and so the physiological function of vascular muscarinic receptors is uncertain.

Choline esters. Carbachol and **bethanechol** are quaternary compounds, that do not penetrate the blood–brain barrier. Their actions are much more prolonged than those of acetylcholine, because they are not hydrolysed by cholinesterase.

Pilocarpine possesses a tertiary N atom which confers increased lipid solubility. This enables the drug to penetrate the cornea readily when applied locally, and enter the brain when given systemically.

Anticholinesterases. These are indirectly acting cholinomimetics. The commonly used anticholinesterase drugs are quaternary compounds that do not pass the blood–brain barrier and have negligible central effects. They are poorly absorbed orally. **Physostigmine** (eserine) is a tertiary amine and is much more lipid soluble. It is well absorbed after oral or local administration (e.g. as eyedrops) and passes into the brain.

Mechanism of action. Initially, acetylcholine binds to the active site of the esterase and is hydrolysed, producing free choline and acetylated enzyme. In a second step, the covalent acetyl–enzyme bond is split with the addition of water. **Edrophonium** is the main example of a reversible anticholinesterase. It binds by electrostatic forces to the active site of the enzyme. It does not form covalent bonds with the enzyme and so is very short acting (2–10 minutes). The carbamate esters (e.g. **neostigmine, pyridostigmine**) undergo the same two-step process as acetylcholine, except that the breakdown of the carbamylated enzyme is much slower (30 minutes to 6 hours). Organophosphorous agents (e.g. **echothiopate**) result in a phosphorylated enzyme active site. The covalent phosphorus–enzyme bond is very stable and the enzyme is inactivated for hundreds of hours. For this reason, the organophosphorous compounds are referred to as irreversible anticholinesterases. They are extremely toxic and used as insecticides (parathion, malathion) and chemical warfare agents.

Effects of anticholinesterases are generally similar to those produced by the directly acting muscarinic agonists, but, in addition, transmission at the neuromuscular junction is potentiated. The cholinesterase inhibitors produce less vasodilatation than the directly acting agonists because they can only act on the (few) vessels possessing cholinergic innervation. Also, stimulation of sympathetic ganglia may oppose the vasodilator effects of the drug. Only large toxic doses of anticholinesterase produce marked bradycardia and hypotension.

Toxic doses initially cause signs of extreme muscarinic stimulation: miosis, salivation, sweating, bronchial constriction, bronchosecretion, vomiting and diarrhoea. Excessive stimulation of nicotinic receptors may cause depolarizing neuromuscular blockade. If the drug is lipid soluble (e.g. physostigmine, organophosphorous compounds), convulsions, coma and respiratory arrest may occur. Strong nucleophiles (e.g. **pralidoxime**) can split the phosphorus–enzyme bond initially formed by organophosphorous compounds and 'regenerate' the enzyme. Later this becomes impossible because a process of 'ageing' strengthens the phosphorus–enzyme bond.

CHOLINERGIC RECEPTOR ANTAGONISTS

Ganglion blockers cause hypotension, mydriasis, dry mouth, anhidrosis, constipation, urinary retention and impotence. Trimetaphan is used to produce controlled hypotension during certain surgical procedures.

Muscarinic antagonists. Atropine occurs in deadly nightshade (*Atropa belladonna*). It is a weak central stimulant, especially on the vagal nucleus, and low doses often cause bradycardia. Higher doses cause tachycardia. **Hyoscine** (*scopolamine*) is more sedative than atropine and often produces drowsiness and amnesia. Toxic doses of both drugs cause excitement, agitation, hallucination and coma. The effects of muscarinic antagonists can be worked out by studying the figure in Chapter 7. The student should understand why these drugs produce dilated pupils, blurred vision, dry mouth, constipation and difficulty with micturition.

9 Drugs acting on the sympathetic system

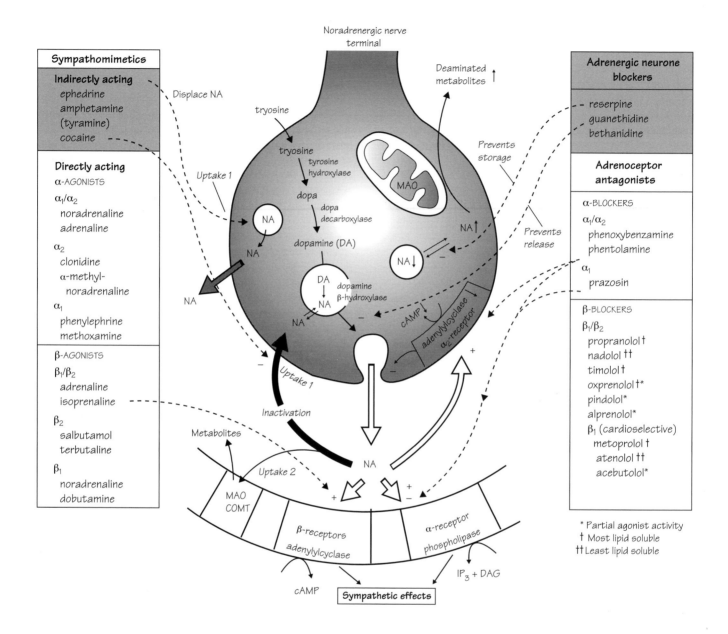

The sympathetic nervous system is important in regulating organs such as the heart and peripheral vasculature (Chapters 15 and 18). The transmitter released from sympathetic nerve endings is noradrenaline (⟶), but in response to some forms of stress adrenaline is also released from the adrenal medulla. These catecholamines are inactivated mainly by **reuptake** (⟶).

Sympathomimetics (left) are drugs that partially or completely mimic the actions of noradrenaline and adrenaline. They act either **directly** on α- and/or β-adrenoceptors (left, open column) or **indirectly** on the presynaptic terminals (top left, shaded), usually by causing the release of noradrenaline (⟶). The effects of adrenoceptor stimulation can be seen in the figure in Chapter 7.

β₂-Adrenoceptor agonists cause bronchial dilatation and are used in

the treatment of asthma (Chapter 11). They are also used to relax uterine muscle in an attempt to prevent preterm labour. **β₁-Adrenoceptor agonists** (dobutamine) are sometimes used to stimulate the force of heart contraction in severe low-output heart failure (Chapter 18). **α₁-Agonists** (e.g. **phenylephrine**) are used as mydriatics (Chapter 10) and in many popular decongestant preparations. **α₂-Agonists**, notably **clonidine** and **methyldopa** (which acts after its conversion to α-methylnoradrenaline, a false transmitter), are centrally acting hypotensive drugs (Chapter 15).

Sympathomimetic amines that act mainly by causing **noradrenaline release** (e.g. **amphetamine**) have the α/β selectivity of noradrenaline. **Ephedrine**, in addition to causing noradrenaline release, also has a direct action. Its effects resemble those of adrenaline, but last much longer. Ephedrine is a mild central stimulant, but amphetamine, which enters the brain more readily, has a much greater stimulant effect on mood and alertness and a depressant effect on appetite. Amphetamine and similar drugs have a high abuse potential and are rarely used (Chapter 31).

β-Adrenoceptor antagonists (β-blockers) (bottom right) are important drugs in the treatment of hypertension (Chapter 15), angina (Chapter 16), cardiac arrhythmias (Chapter 17) and glaucoma (Chapter 10). **α-Adrenoceptor antagonists (α-blockers)** (middle right) have limited clinical applications. **Prazosin**, a selective α_1-antagonist, is sometimes used in the treatment of hypertension. **Phenoxybenzamine**, an

irreversible antagonist, is used to block the α-effects of the large amounts of catecholamines released from tumours of the adrenal medulla (phaeochromocytoma). Many α-blockers have been (and are) used in the treatment of peripheral vascular occlusive disease, usually with little success.

Adrenergic neurone-blocking drugs (top right, shaded) either deplete the nerve terminals of noradrenaline (reserpine) or prevent its release. They were used as hypotensive agents (Chapter 15).

Reuptake of noradrenaline by a high-affinity transport system (Uptake 1) in the nerve terminals 'recaptures' most of the transmitter and is the main method of terminating its effects. A similar (extraneuronal) transport system (Uptake 2) exists in the tissues but is less selective and less easily saturated.

MAO (monoamine oxidase) and COMT (catechol-O-methyltransferase) are widely distributed enzymes that catabolize catecholamines. Inhibition of MAO and COMT has little potentiating effect on responses to sympathetic nerve stimulation or injected catecholamines (noradrenaline, adrenaline) because they are largely inactivated by reuptake.

α_1-Adrenoceptors are postsynaptic. Their activation in several tissues (e.g. smooth muscle, salivary glands) causes an increase in inositol trisphosphate and subsequently cytosolic calcium (Chapter 1), which triggers muscle contraction (except gut) or glandular secretion.

α_2-Adrenoceptors occur on noradrenergic nerve terminals. Their activation by noradrenaline diminishes further transmitter release by a mechanism involving the inhibition of adenylyl cyclase and a reduced Ca^{2+} influx during the action potential.

β-Adrenoceptor activation results in stimulation of adenylyl cyclase, increasing the conversion of ATP to cAMP. The cAMP acts as a 'second messenger' coupling receptor activation response.

SYMPATHOMIMETICS

Indirectly acting sympathomimetics resemble the structure of noradrenaline closely enough to be transported by Uptake 1 into nerve terminals where they displace vesicular noradrenaline into the cytoplasm. Some of the noradrenaline is metabolized by MAO but the remainder is released by carrier-mediated transport to activate adrenoceptors.

Amphetamine is resistant to MAO. Its peripheral actions (e.g. tachycardia, hypertension) and central stimulant actions are mainly due to catecholamine release. D-amphetamine (dexamphetamine) is used in narcolepsy and sometimes in hyperkinetic children. Dependence on amphetamine-like drugs is common (Chapter 31).

Cocaine, in addition to being a local anaesthetic (Chapter 5), is a sympathomimetic because it inhibits the reuptake of noradrenaline by nerve terminals. It has an intense central stimulant effect that has made it a popular drug of abuse (Chapter 31).

Directly acting sympathomimetics. The effect of sympathomimetic drugs in humans depends on their receptor specificity (α and/or β) and on the compensatory reflexes they evoke.

Adrenaline and **noradrenaline** are destroyed in the gut and are short

lasting when injected because of uptake and metabolism. Adrenaline increases the blood pressure by stimulating the rate and force of the heart beat (β_1-effects). Stimulation of vascular α-receptors causes vasoconstriction (viscera, skin) but β_2-stimulation causes vasodilatation (skeletal muscle) and the total peripheral resistance may actually decrease.

Noradrenaline has little or no effect on the vascular β_2-receptors and so the α-mediated vasoconstriction is unopposed. The resulting rise in blood pressure reflexively slows the heart, usually overcoming the direct β_1-stimulant action on heart rate.

Adrenaline by injection has an important use in the treatment of *anaphylactic shock* (Chapter 11).

β-Receptor-selective drugs. Isoprenaline selectively stimulates β-receptors, increasing the rate and force of the heart beat and causing vasodilatation. These effects result in a fall in diastolic and mean arterial pressure with little change in systolic pressure.

β_2-Adrenoceptor agonists are relatively selective drugs that produce bronchodilatation at doses that cause minimal effects on the heart. They are resistant to MAO and are probably not taken up into neurones. Their main use is in the treatment of asthma (Chapter 11).

ADRENOCEPTOR ANTAGONISTS

α-Blockers reduce arteriolar and venous tone, causing a fall in peripheral resistance and hypotension (Chapter 15). They reverse the pressor effects of adrenaline because its β_2-mediated vasodilator effects are unopposed by α-mediated vasoconstriction and the peripheral resistance falls (adrenaline reversal). α-Blockers cause a reflex tachycardia, which is greater with non-selective drugs that also block α_2-presynaptic receptors on the heart because the augmented release of noradrenaline stimulates further the cardiac β-receptors. **Prazosin**, a selective α_1-antagonist, causes relatively little tachycardia.

β-Blockers vary in their *lipid solubility* and *cardioselectivity*. However, they all block β_1-receptors and are equally effective in reducing blood pressure and preventing angina. The more lipid-soluble drugs are more rapidly absorbed from the gut, undergo more first-pass hepatic metabolism and are more rapidly eliminated. They are also more likely to enter the brain and cause central effects (e.g. bad dreams). *Cardioselectivity* is only relative and diminishes with higher doses. Nevertheless, selective β_1-blockade seems to produce less peripheral vasoconstriction (cold hands and feet) and does not reduce the response to exercise-induced hypoglycaemia (stimulation of gluconeogenesis in the liver is mediated by β_2-receptors). Cardioselective drugs may have sufficient β_2-activity to precipitate severe bronchospasm in patients with asthma and they should avoid β-blockers. Some β-blockers possess *intrinsic sympathomimetic activity* (i.e. are partial agonists, Chapter 2). The clinical importance of this is debatable, but see Chapter 16.

10 Ocular pharmacology

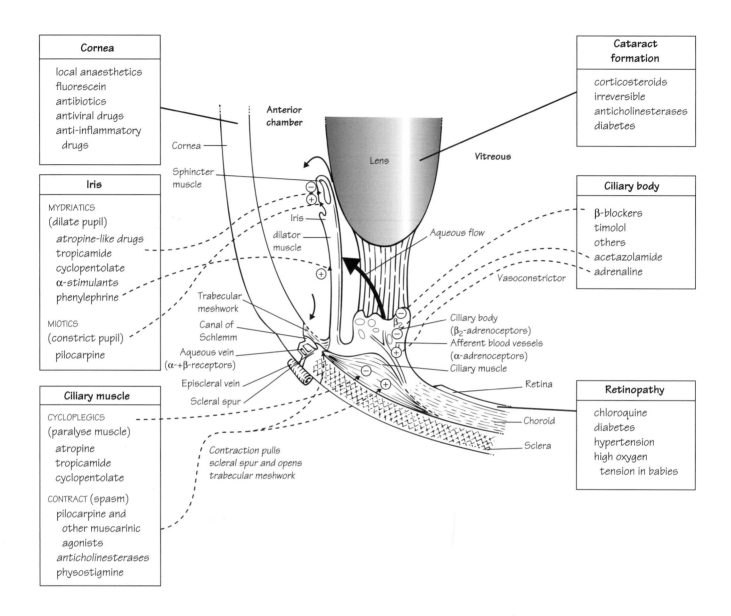

Cornea

local anaesthetics
fluorescein
antibiotics
antiviral drugs
anti-inflammatory
drugs

Iris

MYDRIATICS
(dilate pupil)
atropine-like drugs
tropicamide
cyclopentolate
α-stimulants
phenylephrine

MIOTICS
(constrict pupil)
pilocarpine

Ciliary muscle

CYCLOPLEGICS
(paralyse muscle)
atropine
tropicamide
cyclopentolate

CONTRACT (spasm)
pilocarpine and
other muscarinic
agonists
anticholinesterases
physostigmine

Cataract formation

corticosteroids
irreversible
anticholinesterases
diabetes

Ciliary body

β-blockers
timolol
others
acetazolamide
adrenaline

Retinopathy

chloroquine
diabetes
hypertension
high oxygen
tension in babies

Anterior chamber
Cornea
Sphincter muscle
Iris
dilator muscle
Trabecular meshwork
Canal of Schlemm
Aqueous vein (α-+β-receptors)
Episcleral vein
Scleral spur
Contraction pulls scleral spur and opens trabecular meshwork

Lens
Vitreous
Aqueous flow
Vasoconstrictor
Ciliary body (β₂-adrenoceptors)
Afferent blood vessels (α-adrenoceptors)
Ciliary muscle
Retina
Choroid
Sclera

The eye is an inflated spherical shell, its outer layer being the tough, collagen-rich sclera. The normal **intraocular pressure** (IOP) is about 15 mmHg and is maintained by a balance of aqueous humour formation by the *ciliary body* (➡) and outflow through the *trabecular meshwork* into the canal of Schlemm ( ). In open-angle **glaucoma** the IOP remains above 24 mmHg because pathological changes in the trabecular meshwork decrease the outflow of aqueous. Since the elevated IOP will eventually damage the optic nerve, the pressure is reduced, usually with drugs. This can be done either by increasing aqueous outflow with **muscarinic agonists**, such as **pilocarpine** (bottom left), or by reducing aqueous formation with a variety of drugs (middle right) but especially **timolol**, a β-blocker.

At the front of the eye, the sclera runs into the **cornea** (top left) whose transparency is obtained by alignment of the collagen fibres. Many superficial manipulations such as tonometry (measurement of the intraocular pressure) and the removal of corneal foreign bodies require the instillation of a *local anaesthetic*. **Fluorescein** is common-ly instilled into the eye to reveal damaged areas of corneal epithelium, which are stained bright green by the dye. **Inflammation** of the cornea resulting from allergy or chemical burns is treated with topical anti-inflammatory drugs (Chapter 33). Infections are not treated with anti-inflammatory agents except together with an effective chemotherapeutic agent. This is because anti-inflammatory drugs reduce resistance to invading micro-organisms.

The **iris** (middle left) possesses a sphincter muscle, which receives parasympathetic nerves, and a dilator muscle, which is innervated by sympathetic fibres. Thus, muscarinic antagonists and α-adrenoceptor agonists *dilate* the pupil (**mydriasis**), whilst muscarinic agonists and α-adrenoceptor antagonists *constrict* the pupil (**miosis**).

Contraction of the parasympathetically innervated **ciliary muscle** (bottom left) allows the lens to become thicker and accommodation for near vision occurs. Thus, muscarinic antagonists *paralyse* the ciliary muscle (**cycloplegia**) and prevent accommodation for near vision, whilst agonists cause accommodation and a loss of far vision.

The **lens** (middle top) provides the adjustable part of the eye's refractive power. Opacity of the lens is called a cataract. Some drugs, notably corticosteroids, may cause cataracts.

The retina is a part of the central nervous system but it seems little affected by drugs, probably because of the effective blood–retinal barrier. The retina may occasionally be damaged by drugs (e.g. chloroquine, quinine, ethambutol) or by high oxygen tension in newborn babies.

Ciliary body. The processes of the ciliary body are highly vascularized and are the sites of aqueous humour formation. The ciliary epithelial cells, which contain ATPase and carbonic anhydrase, absorb Na^+ selectively from the stroma and transport it into the intercellular clefts, which open only on the aqueous humour side. The hyperosmolality in the clefts causes water flow from the stroma, producing a continuous flow of aqueous. The ciliary epithelium is leaky, allowing significant passive filtration, and up to 30% of aqueous may be formed by ultrafiltration.

Trabecular meshwork. The aqueous humour circulates through the pupil and is drained into the canal of Schlemm, which is a circular gutter within the surface of the sclera at the limbus. The sieve-like trabecular meshwork is the roof of the gutter, through which the aqueous must pass before it is eventually drained away into the episcleral veins.

GLAUCOMA

This is a group of ocular diseases with the common features of abnormally high IOP and ultimate loss of vision if untreated. It occurs in about 1% of people over 40 years of age. Viewed through an ophthalmoscope, the optic disc appears depressed (cupping) because of the loss of nerve fibres. The mechanism by which the nerve fibres are destroyed in glaucoma is unclear, but may involve mechanical factors and/or local ischaemia. Open-angle (chronic simple) glaucoma is the most common form of the disease. In closed-angle glaucoma, the angle between the cornea and the iris is abnormally small. Occasionally, the angle closes completely, preventing aqueous outflow, and the IOP quickly rises. Since permanent damage to the retina can occur during these attacks, the pressure must be reduced as quickly as possible by intensive instillation of pilocarpine eyedrops combined, if necessary, with intravenous *acetazolamide* and intravenous hypertonic mannitol (an osmotic agent), to remove water. Acetazolamide inhibits carbonic anhydrase in the ciliary body and prevents bicarbonate synthesis. This leads to a fall in sodium transport and aqueous formation because bicarbonate and sodium transport are linked.

Pilocarpine, being a tertiary amine, diffuses readily through the cornea into the aqueous humour. It reduces the IOP by contracting the ciliary muscle. This pulls the scleral spur and results in the trabecular meshwork being stretched and separated. The fluid pathways are opened up and aqueous outflow is increased.

Physostigmine is rarely used in glaucoma because of contact sensitivity reactions. Irreversible anticholinesterases, such as echothiopate, are associated with a high degree of cataract formation.

All parasympathomimetics cause miosis, resulting in poor night vision and complaints of 'dimming of vision'. Accommodation spasm that increases near-sightedness causing blurred vision is not usually a problem in the age group that develops glaucoma. Some patients find these effects intolerable.

β-Blockers. Timolol is the drug of choice in open-angle glaucoma. It blocks $β_2$-adrenoceptors on the ciliary processes and so reduces aqueous secretion. In addition, timolol may block β-receptors in the afferent blood vessels supplying the ciliary processes. The resulting vasoconstriction results in reduced ultrafiltration and aqueous formation. Timolol avoids the unpleasant effects of pilocarpine on the eye, but it is absorbed systemically and may provoke bronchospasm in asthmatics or bradycardia in susceptible patients. Therefore, β-blockers (even selective $β_1$-antagonists) should be avoided in patients with asthma, heart failure, heart block or bradycardia.

Adrenaline and α-adrenoceptor stimulants lower the IOP by an α-mediated vasoconstriction of the ciliary body afferent blood vessels. Confusingly, α-antagonists and β-adrenoceptor agonists (especially $β_2$-stimulants) also lower the IOP. These drugs increase the outflow of aqueous rather than reducing its formation, presumably by dilatation of the aqueous veins and/or episcleral veins. **Guanethidine** increases and prolongs the actions of adrenaline by blocking its uptake by the tissues.

Laser trabecular surgery may be used as an alternative to drugs in glaucoma. Under local anaesthesia, the surgeon uses an argon or diode laser to place about 100 evenly spaced lesions on the inner surface of the trabecular meshwork. The laser 'burns' cause localized shrinkage, which exerts tension on the adjacent, untreated tissue, opening spaces in the meshwork and allowing increased aqueous drainage. In closed-angle glaucoma, a YAG (yttrium aluminium garnet) laser may be used to make a hole at the periphery of the iris. This prevents the forward movement of the iris that precipitates acute glaucoma and is usually due to a partial block of aqueous flow through the pupil.

Whilst the benefits of treating patients with closed-angle glaucoma are clear, the same cannot be said for patients with open-angle glaucoma, because the available evidence does not convincingly show that treatment with drugs or laser surgery affects the long-term progress of the disease.

MYDRIATICS

Mydriasis (dilatation of the pupil) is required for ophthalmoscopy. The drops most commonly used are the relatively short-acting muscarinic antagonists **tropicamide** and **cyclopentolate**, which produce both mydriasis and cycloplegia. The α-adrenoceptor stimulant **phenylephrine** may be used to produce mydriasis without affecting the pupillary light reflex or accommodation. When the examination is complete, **physostigmine** or **pilocarpine** eyedrops can be given to antagonize the mydriatic, but this is only done very rarely. Phenylephrine mydriasis can be reversed with the α-antagonist, **thymoxamine**. Mydriasis may precipitate acute closed-angle glaucoma in susceptible patients who are usually aged over 60 years.

11 Asthma, hay fever and anaphylaxis

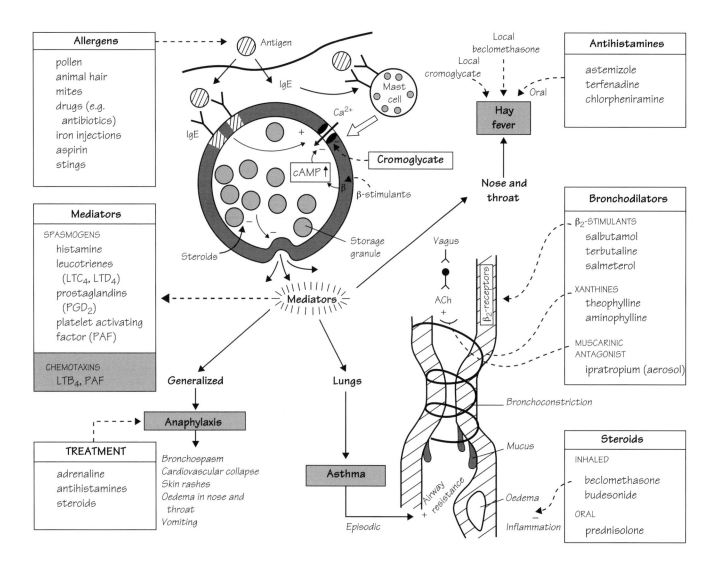

Asthma, hay fever and anaphylaxis (shaded boxes) are caused by the same basic processes: *IgE* antibody attaches to mast cells (top left), and on renewed exposure to the same antigen (⊘) degranulation of the mast cells occurs with the production and release of **mediators** (middle left). If the release of mediators is localized, hay fever (top right) or asthma (bottom right) result, but a massive general release causes anaphylaxis, which is a rare, but life-threatening, reaction to bee stings and penicillin or other drugs. Antigens that can trigger these reactions are called **allergens** (top left).

Bronchial asthma is an inflammatory disease in which the calibre of the airways is chronically narrowed by oedema and is unstable. During an attack the patient suffers from wheezing and difficulty in breathing due to bronchospasm, mucosal oedema and mucus formation (bottom right). Eventually the chronic inflammation causes irreversible changes to the airways (bottom right). When the acute attack has an allergic basis the term *extrinsic asthma* is often used. When there is no obvious allergic basis for the disease it is called *intrinsic asthma*.

In **mild to moderate asthma** the first-line drugs are short-acting β_2-adrenoceptor agonists (β_2-stimulants, middle right) inhaled from pres-surized containers when required. If β-agonists are required more than once a day, then regular administration of inhaled steroid or cromoglycate is added (bottom right). In more severe asthma, short-acting β-agonists are retained with the addition of high-dose inhaled steroids and, if necessary, a second-line drug, e.g. inhaled salmeterol, inhaled ipratropium (a muscarinic antagonist), oral sustained release theophylline. Some patients are controlled only by oral steroids (usually *prednisolone*, Chapter 33).

Acute severe attacks of asthma (status asthmaticus) which are not controlled by the patient's usual drugs are potentially fatal and must be dealt with as an emergency, requiring hospital admission.

Anaphylaxis (bottom left) requires prompt treatment with **adrenaline** (Chapter 9), given by intramuscular injection that is repeated every 10 minutes until the blood pressure and pulse improve. Antihistamines (e.g. chlorpheniramine) given intravenously after the adrenaline are useful but corticosteroids take several hours to produce beneficial effects.

Hay fever is most commonly caused by allergy to grass pollen. **Anti-histamines** control some symptoms and nasal corticosteroids are very effective. Cromoglycate eye drops may be a valuable adjunct in allergic conjunctivitis.

IgE is the major class of reaginic antibody. In allergic patients, specific antibody levels may be increased to 100 times greater than normal. Binding of the F_c portion of the antibody to receptors on mast cells, followed by cross-linking of adjacent molecules by antigen, triggers degranulation by a mechanism involving Ca^{2+} influx.

Mast cells contain the body stores of histamine and occur in almost all tissues. Within the mast cells, histamine is bound with heparin and ATP in cytoplasmic granules. Histamine release normally involves an influx of Ca^{2+} ions and, because the permeability of the cell membrane to Ca^{2+} ions is reduced when intracellular cAMP levels are raised, drugs that either stimulate cAMP synthesis (β_2-adrenoceptor agonists) or prevent its breakdown (xanthines) reduce histamine release.

Mediators. The initial phase of an asthma attack is due mainly to spasm of the bronchial smooth muscle caused by the release of *spasmogens* (middle left) from mast cells. In many asthmatics, a second delayed phase results from the release of chemotaxins (centre left, shaded) which attract inflammatory cells, especially eosinophils. These inflammatory processes cause *vasodilatation, oedema, mucus secretion* and *bronchospasm* and are at first reversible. However, permanent damage to the bronchial epithelium and smooth muscle hypertrophy eventually lead to irreversible airways obstruction. This damage seems to be caused mainly by substances released from the eosinophil granules (especially eosinophil major basic protein and granule peroxidase).

BRONCHODILATORS

β-Adrenoceptor stimulants. The airway smooth muscle has few adrenergic nerve fibres but many β_2-receptors, stimulation of which causes bronchodilatation. Activation of β_2-adrenoceptors relaxes smooth muscle by increasing intracellular cAMP which activates a protein kinase. This inhibits muscle contraction by phosphorylating and inhibiting myosin-light-chain kinase. β_2-Agonists such as **salbutamol** are usually given by inhalation. They are not specific, but β_1 effects (cardiac stimulation) are not usually seen at doses which cause bronchodilatation. Adverse effects include fine tremor, nervous tension and tachycardia, but these are not usually troublesome when the drug is given by inhalation. Oral administration is usually restricted to children and other patients who cannot use an aerosol preparation. **Salmeterol** is much longer lasting than salbutamol, but has a slower onset and is not intended for symptomatic relief. There is some evidence that inhaled β_2-agonists given regularly, rather than 'as necessary', cause asthma to deteriorate but it is not known why.

Ipratropium is a muscarinic antagonist and a moderately effective bronchodilator, presumably because it reduces reflex vagal bronchoconstriction which results from histamine stimulation of sensory (irritant) receptors in the airways. Ipratropium given by inhalation rarely causes atropine-like side effects.

Xanthines. Theophylline may benefit children who cannot use inhalants, and adults with predominantly nocturnal symptoms. Theophylline often cause adverse effects, even oral sustained-release theophylline preparations which are effective for up to 12 hours. Even when plasma concentrations are in the therapeutic range (10–20 mg l⁻¹), nausea, headache, insomnia and abdominal discomfort are common.

Above 25 mg l⁻¹, toxic effects include serious arrhythmias and convulsions that may be fatal. It is not known how theophylline causes bronchodilatation in asthmatics. Theophylline inhibits phosphodiesterase and increases cellular cAMP levels. The concentration of theophylline that inhibits most phosphodiesterases is higher than the therapeutic range but there is some evidence that a subtype of the enzyme in airway smooth muscle is more sensitive to the drug.

CROMOGLYCATE

This is a prophylactic drug and is of no value in acute attacks. It has anti-inflammatory actions in some patients (especially children) but it is not possible to predict which patients will benefit. Cromoglycate must be given regularly and it may be several weeks before beneficial effects are apparent. The mechanism of action of cromoglycate is unclear. It may act by decreasing the sensitivity of bronchial sensory nerves, abolishing local reflexes that stimulate inflammation.

GLUCOCORTICOIDS

Steroids effectively increase the airway calibre in asthma by reducing bronchial inflammatory reactions (e.g. oedema and mucus hypersecretion) and by modifying allergic reactions. Oral administration of steroids is associated with many serious adverse effects (Chapter 33) but, except for high doses, these can be avoided in asthma by aerosol administration of the drugs (e.g. **beclomethasone**). Inhaled steroids are usually effective in 3–7 days, but oral steroids may be necessary in some patients, where all other therapy fails. Steroid nasal sprays (e.g. **beclomethasone, budesonide**) are very effective in hay fever and are especially useful in patients with nasal congestion that is not affected by antihistamines.

ACUTE SEVERE ASTHMA

Oxygen is given together with nebulized or intravenous β_2-agonists (e.g. **salbutamol**). Then intravenous **hydrocortisone** is given, but this will not be effective for several hours (Chapter 33). Nebulized **ipratropium** may also be used if required, but may cause difficulty in micturition. If these drugs do not produce a response, an intravenous infusion of aminophylline may help but there is little evidence that it does. Artificial ventilation may be required.

ANTIHISTAMINES

Antagonists that block H_1-histamine receptors are used in the treatment of allergic conditions such as hay fever, urticaria, drug sensitivity rashes, pruritis and insect bites and stings. Older antihistamine drugs (e.g. **chlorpheniramine, trimeprazine, promethazine**) have antimuscarinic actions and pass the blood–brain barrier, commonly causing drowsiness and psychomotor impairment. Newer agents (e.g. **astemizole, terfenadine**) do not have atropine-like actions and because they do not cross the blood–brain barrier to any extent, they do not cause psychomotor impairment. However, they may be less effective. Terfenadine and astemizole rarely cause cardiac arrhythmias. They should not be given concomitantly with other proarrhythmic drugs, e.g. tricyclics, antidepressants, antipsychotics, anti-arrhythmics.

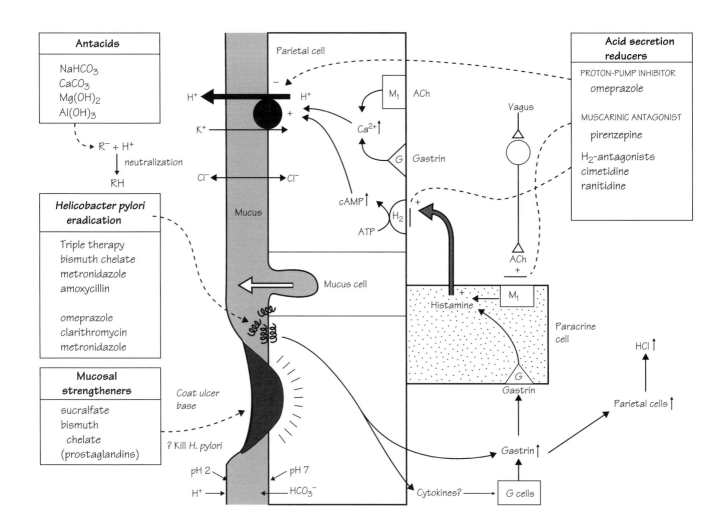

The term **peptic ulcer** refers to any ulcer in an area where the mucosa is bathed in the hydrochloric acid and pepsin of gastric juice (i.e. the stomach and upper part of the duodenum). Drugs that are effective in the treatment of peptic ulcer either **reduce gastric acid secretion** (right) or **increase mucosal resistance** to acid–pepsin attack (bottom left).

Acid secretion from the *parietal cells* (■▶) is reduced by **H_2-histamine antagonists** (right), which are the first-line drugs in ulcer treatment. **Omeprazole** can produce virtual anacidity by irreversibly inhibiting the proton pump (●), which transports H^+ ions out of the parietal cells. It is very effective in promoting ulcer healing, even in patients who are resistant to H_2-antagonists. **Pirenzepine**, a cholinergic M_1-muscarinic antagonist with a relatively selective action in the gut, also decreases acid secretion, but less effectively than the H_2-blockers and is little used. The 'mucosal strengtheners' (bottom left) increase ulcer healing by binding to the ulcer base (left, ■). This provides **physical protection** and allows the secretion of HCO_3^- to re-establish the pH gradient normally present in the mucus layer (▨) that originates from mucus-secreting cells (⇨).

Peptic ulcers, however healed, will often recur without continuous drug administration. There is evidence that the recurrence of ulcers is slower following bismuth chelate administration, but the reason for this is unknown. It may well be due to the antibacterial action of bismuth, because chronic infection of the stomach with *Helicobacter pylori* (ᗃᗂ) is now thought to be an important aetiological factor in ulcer formation. *H. pylori* infection results in a chronic hypergastrinaemia which stimulates acid production and causes ulcers (bottom, right). Eradication of *H. pylori* requires a combination of antibiotics (left, centre) but, when successful, there seems to be a much reduced chance of the ulcer recurring.

Antacids (top left) are bases that raise the gastric luminal pH by neutralizing gastric acid (middle left). They provide effective treatment for many dyspepsias and symptomatic relief in peptic ulcer and oesophageal reflux. Many proprietary mixtures which usually contain magnesium or aluminium salts are available.

ACID SECRETION

Parietal cells secrete acid into the stomach lumen. This is achieved by a unique H^+/K^+ ATPase (proton pump) which catalyses the exchange of intracellular H^+ for extracellular K^+. The secretion of HCl is stimulated by *acetylcholine* (ACh), released from vagal postganglionic fibres (right of figure) and *gastrin*, released into the bloodstream from G-cells in the antral mucosa when they detect amino acids and peptides (from food) in the stomach, and by gastric distension via local and long reflexes.

Although the parietal cells possess muscarinic (M_1) and gastrin receptors (G), both acetylcholine and gastrin mainly stimulate acid secretion indirectly, by releasing *histamine* from paracrine cells (right, ▦) located close to the parietal cells. Histamine then acts locally (⬅) on the parietal cells, where activation of histamine H_2-receptors (H_2) results in an increase in intracellular cAMP and the secretion of acid. Because acetylcholine and gastrin act indirectly by releasing histamine, the effects on acid secretion of both vagal stimulation and gastrin are reduced by H_2-receptor antagonists.

Cholinergic agonists can powerfully stimulate acid secretion in the presence of H_2-antagonists, indicating that ACh released from the vagus must have limited access to the parietal cell muscarinic receptors. Gastrin acting directly on the parietal cells has a weak effect on acid secretion, but this is greatly potentiated when the histamine receptors are activated.

PROTECTIVE FACTORS

Mucus layer. This forms a physical barrier (approximately $500\,\mu m$ thick) on the surface of the stomach and proximal duodenum, and consists of a mucus gel into which HCO_3^- is secreted. Within the gel matrix the HCO_3^- neutralizes acid diffusing from the lumen. This creates a pH gradient and the gastric mucosa is maintained at a neutral pH, even when the stomach contents are at pH 2. Prostaglandins E_2 and I_2 are synthesized by the gastric mucosa, where they are thought to exert a cytoprotective action by stimulating the secretion of mucus and bicarbonate, and by increasing the mucosal blood flow.

ULCER HEALING DRUGS

Acid-secretion reducers

Histamine H_2-receptor antagonists. **Cimetidine** and **ranitidine** are rapidly absorbed orally. They block the action of histamine on the parietal cells and reduce acid secretion. These drugs relieve the pain of peptic ulcer and increase the rate of ulcer healing. The incidence of side effects is low. Cimetidine has slight anti-androgenic actions, and rarely causes gynaecomastia. Cimetidine also binds to cytochrome P-450 and may reduce the hepatic metabolism of drugs (e.g. warfarin, phenytoin and theophylline).

Proton-pump inhibitors. **Omeprazole** is inactive at neutral pH, but in acid it rearranges into two types of reactive molecule which react with sulphydryl groups in the H^+/K^+ ATPase (proton pump) responsible for transporting H^+ ions out of the parietal cells. Since the enzyme is irreversibly inhibited, acid secretion only resumes after the synthesis of new enzyme. It is particularly useful in patients with severe gastric acid hypersecretion due to Zollinger–Ellison syndrome, a rare condition caused by an islet-cell gastrin-secreting tumour of the pancreas, and in patients with reflux oesophagitis where severe ulceration is usually resistant to other drugs.

H. pylori is a mobile spiral-shaped Gram-negative rod found deep in the mucus layer where a pH of 7.0 is optimal for its growth. The bacteria invade the epithelial cell surface to some extent and toxins and ammonia produced by strong urease activity may damage the cells. Gastritis associated with *H. pylori* infection persists for years, or for life, and is associated with a sustained increase in gastrin release, which increases the basal release of HCl. The increased gastrin release may be due to cytokines resulting from inflammation, which also compromises mucosal defence. A trophic effect of the hypergastrinaemia increases the mass of the parietal cells causing an exaggerated acid-secreting response to gastrin. In the duodenum, the acid induces mucosal injury and metaplastic cells of the gastric phenotype. Chronic inflammation of these cells leads to ulceration. Eradication of *H. pylori* significantly reduces HCl secretion and heals duodenal, and probably gastric, ulcers. **'Standard triple therapy'** includes bismuth, metronidazole and amoxycillin (for 2 weeks). This regimen eradicates *H. pylori* in about 70–80% of patients but side effects are frequent (nausea, diarrhoea). Omeprazole, clarithromycin and metronidazole eradicates *H. pylori* in 95–100% of patients in 1 week with fewer side effects. Metronidazole resistance may be an increasing problem.

Mucosal strengtheners. Bismuth chelate may act in a similar way to sucralfate. It has a strong affinity for mucosal glycoproteins, especially in the necrotic tissue of the ulcer craters, which become coated in a protective layer of polymer–glycoprotein complex. **Sucralfate** polymerizes below pH 4 to give a very sticky gel that adheres strongly to the base of ulcer craters. Bismuth may blacken the teeth and stools. Bismuth and sucralfate must be given on an empty stomach or they will complex with food proteins.

ANTACIDS

Antacids raise the luminal pH of the stomach. This increases the rate of emptying and so the effect of antacids is short. Gastrin release is increased and because this stimulates acid release, larger amounts of antacids are needed than would be predicted (acid rebound). Frequent high doses of antacids promote ulcer healing, but such treatment is rarely practical.

Sodium bicarbonate is the only useful water-soluble antacid. It acts rapidly but has a transient action and absorbed bicarbonate in high doses may cause systemic alkalosis.

Magnesium hydroxide and magnesium trisilicate are insoluble in water and have a fairly rapid action. Magnesium has a laxative effect and may cause diarrhoea.

Aluminium hydroxide has a relatively slower action. Al^{3+} ions form complexes with certain drugs (e.g. tetracyclines) and tend to cause constipation. Mixtures of magnesium and aluminium compounds may be used to minimize the effects on motility.

13 Drugs acting on the gastrointestinal tract. II: Motility and secretions

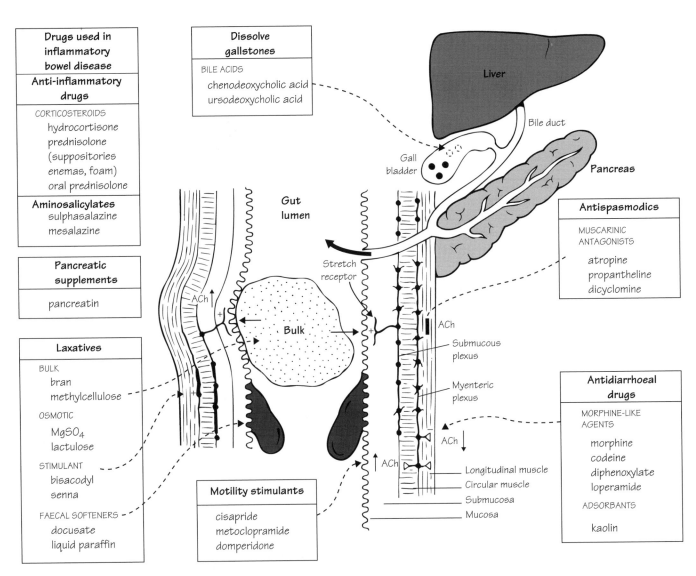

Drugs used in inflammatory bowel disease
Anti-inflammatory drugs
CORTICOSTEROIDS
hydrocortisone
prednisolone
(suppositories enemas, foam)
oral prednisolone
Aminosalicylates
sulphasalazine
mesalazine

Pancreatic supplements
pancreatin

Laxatives
BULK
bran
methylcellulose
OSMOTIC
MgSO$_4$
lactulose
STIMULANT
bisacodyl
senna
FAECAL SOFTENERS
docusate
liquid paraffin

Dissolve gallstones
BILE ACIDS
chenodeoxycholic acid
ursodeoxycholic acid

Motility stimulants
cisapride
metoclopramide
domperidone

Antispasmodics
MUSCARINIC ANTAGONISTS
atropine
propantheline
dicyclomine

Antidiarrhoeal drugs
MORPHINE-LIKE AGENTS
morphine
codeine
diphenoxylate
loperamide
ADSORBANTS
kaolin

Liver — Bile duct — Gall bladder — Pancreas — Gut lumen — Stretch receptor — ACh — Bulk — Submucous plexus — Myenteric plexus — ACh — Longitudinal muscle — Circular muscle — Submucosa — Mucosa

Muscular contractions of the gut and secretion of acid and enzymes are under autonomic control. The enteric part of the autonomic nervous system consists of ganglionated plexuses (–◆–◆–) with complex interconnections supplying the smooth muscle, mucosa and blood vessels. The ganglia (🌣) (parasympathetic) receive extrinsic excitatory fibres from the vagus and inhibitory sympathetic fibres.

Cholinomimetic drugs (e.g. **carbachol, neostigmine**) increase motility and may cause colic and diarrhoea. They are very occasionally used in the treatment of paralytic ileus (Chapter 8). More useful **motility stimulants** (bottom middle) facilitate acetylcholine release from the myenteric plexus and are used in the treatment of oesophageal reflux and gastric stasis. **Laxatives** (bottom left) are drugs used to increase the motility of the gut and encourage defaecation. **Bulk** (⠿) laxatives stimulate stretch receptors in the mucosa. **Stimulant laxatives** stimulate the myenteric plexus, and some drugs act as *lubricants* (▮).

Muscarinic antagonists (top right) reduce gastrointestinal motility and are used to reduce spasm in irritable bowel syndrome (antispasmodics). Antidiarrhoeal drugs (bottom right) include antimotility drugs, but replacement of water and electrolyte loss is generally more important than drug treatment, especially in infants and in infectious diarrhoea.

Anti-inflammatory corticosteroids and aminosalicylates (top left) are used in ulcerative colitis and Crohn's disease. To reduce the need for systemic steroids it is usual to add **azathioprine**, an immunosuppressant (Chapter 43).

In the duodenum, bile from the liver (top right) and pancreatic juice from the pancreas (right, ▭) enter (➡) usually through a common opening that is restricted by the sphincter of Oddi. **Bile acids** (top middle) are sometimes used to dissolve cholesterol gallstones (●). **Pancreatic supplements** (left middle) are given orally when the secretion of pancreatic juice is absent or reduced.

MOTILITY STIMULANTS

Metoclopramide and **domperidone** are dopamine antagonists and by blocking central dopamine receptors in the chemoreceptor trigger zone they produce an antinausea/antiemetic action (see also Chapter 30). The drugs also increase contractions in the stomach and enhance the tone of the lower oesophageal sphincter, actions that combine to speed the transit of contents from the stomach. The prokinetic actions of metoclopramide and domperidone result from the facilitation of acetylcholine release from the myenteric plexus rather than by dopamine antagonism. **Cisapride** also increases gut motility by facilitating acetylcholine release but it does not have dopamine antagonist activity and is not an antiemetic.

LAXATIVES

Constipation is characterized by abdominal discomfort, loss of appetite and malaise resulting from insufficient frequency of defaecation; this results in abnormally hard and dry faeces. The frequency and volume of defaecation are best regulated by diet, but drugs may be needed for specific purposes (e.g. before surgery of the colon or rectum).

Bulk laxatives increase the volume of the intestinal contents, stimulating peristalsis. They include indigestible polysaccharides such as cellulose (bran) and methylcellulose. **Osmotic laxatives** increase bulk in the bowel by retaining water by an osmotic effect. They include **lactulose** and salts containing poorly absorbed ions (e.g. $MgSO_4$, Epsom salts).

Stimulant laxatives increase motility by acting on the mucosa or nerve plexuses, which may be damaged by prolonged drug use. They often cause abdominal cramp. **Anthraquinones** are released from precursor glycosides present in **senna** and **cascara**. They stimulate the myenteric plexus. Bisacodyl may act by stimulating sensory nerve endings.

Faecal softeners promote defaecation by softening (e.g. **docusate**) and/or lubricating (e.g. **liquid paraffin**) faeces and assisting evacuation. Chronic use of liquid paraffin may impair absorption of the fat-soluble vitamins A and D and cause paraffinomas.

ANTIDIARRHOEAL DRUGS

Infectious diarrhoea is a very common cause of illness and results in a high mortality in developing countries. Bacterial pathogens cause the most severe forms of infectious diarrhoea, but more often diarrhoea is caused by a viral infection.

Antimotility drugs are widely used to provide symptomatic relief in mild to moderate forms of acute diarrhoea. Opioids such as *morphine*, *diphenoxylate* and *codeine* activate μ-receptors on myenteric neurones and cause hyperpolarization by increasing their potassium conductance. This inhibits acetylcholine release from the myenteric plexus and reduces bowel motility. **Loperamide** is the most appropriate opioid for local effects on the gut because it does not easily penetrate to the brain. Hence, it has few central actions and is unlikely to cause dependence.

Adsorbants such as **kaolin**, either alone or with other drugs, are popular remedies for diarrhoeal illnesses, but there is little evidence that they do any good.

Rehydration therapy. Oral solutions containing electrolytes and glucose are given to correct the severe dehydration that can be caused by infection with toxigenic organisms.

Antibiotics are useful only in certain specific infections, e.g. cholera and severe bacillary dysentry, which are treated with tetracycline. The quinolones (Chapter 37) are more recent agents that seem to be effective against most important diarrhoeal pathogens.

DRUGS USED IN INFLAMMATORY BOWEL DISEASE

Inflammatory bowel disease is divided into two types:
1 **Crohn's disease**, which can affect the entire gut; and
2 **ulcerative colitis**, which affects only the large bowel.
Local or systemic anti-inflammatory **corticosteroids**, e.g. **prednisolone** (Chapter 33), are the main drugs used for acute attacks, but their serious adverse effects make them unsuitable for maintenance treatment. However, oral **budesonide** (slow release) is a corticosteroid with reduced absorption and may not cause adrenal suppression. **Aminosalicylates** reduce the symptoms in mild disease and maintenance treatment reduces the relapse rates of patients in remission. **Sulphasalazine** is a combination of 5-aminosalicylic acid with a sulphonamide. The molecule is cleaved in the colon by bacteria, releasing **5-aminosalicylic acid**, which is the active moiety, and sulphapyridine, which is absorbed and may produce the adverse effects characteristic of sulphonamides (e.g. nausea, rashes, blood disorders) (see Chapter 35). Newer, less toxic drugs are **mesalazine**, which is 5-aminosalicylate in a preparation that releases the drug in the colon, and **olsalazine** (azodisalicylate), which consists of two molecules of 5-aminosalicylic acid joined by an azo bond, cleaved by bacteria in the colon. The mechanism of action of 5-aminosalicylate is unknown.

DRUGS USED TO DISSOLVE GALLSTONES

Bile contains cholesterol and bile salts, the latter being important in keeping cholesterol in solution. An increase in cholesterol concentration or a decrease in bile salts may result in the formation of cholesterol stones. If they give rise to symptoms, laparoscopic cholecystectomy is the treatment of choice. However, small non-calcified stones may be dissolved by prolonged oral administration of the bile acids **chenodeoxycholic** or **ursodeoxycholic acid**, which decrease the cholesterol content of bile by inhibiting an enzyme involved in cholesterol formation. Chenodeoxycholic acid often causes diarrhoea and sometimes liver abnormalities.

PANCREATIC SUPPLEMENTS

Pancreatic juice contains important enzymes that break down proteins (trypsin, chymotrypsin), starch (amylase) and fats (lipase). In some diseases (e.g. chronic pancreatitis and cystic fibrosis) there is an absence or reduction in these enzymes. Patients with pancreatic insufficiency are given **pancreatin**, an extract of pancreas containing protease, lipase and amylase. Because the enzymes are inactivated by gastric acid, it is usual to give an H_2-receptor antagonist (e.g. *cimetidine*) beforehand. Newer enteric-coated preparations that deliver more of the enzymes to the duodenum are available.

14 Drugs acting on the kidney—diuretics

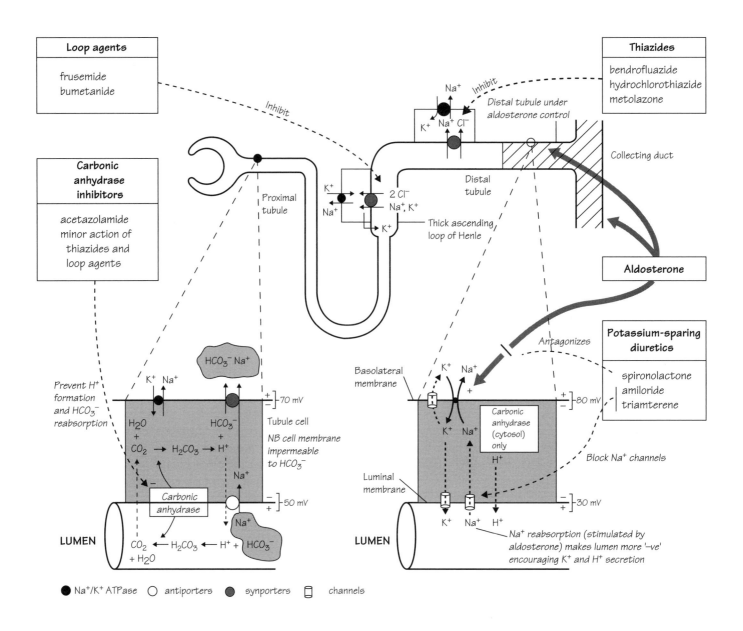

Loop agents

frusemide
bumetanide

Thiazides

bendrofluazide
hydrochlorothiazide
metolazone

Carbonic anhydrase inhibitors

acetazolamide
minor action of thiazides and loop agents

Aldosterone

Potassium-sparing diuretics

spironolactone
amiloride
triamterene

Inhibit

Na^+

Inhibit

Distal tubule under aldosterone control

Collecting duct

K^+ Na^+ Cl^-

Proximal tubule

K^+

$2\,Cl^-$
Na^+, K^+

Na^+

K^+

Distal tubule

Thick ascending loop of Henle

Antagonizes

Prevent H^+ formation and HCO_3^- reabsorption

HCO_3^- Na^+

K^+ Na^+

$-70\ mV$

H_2O
$+$
$CO_2 \rightarrow H_2CO_3 \rightarrow H^+$

HCO_3^-
$+$
H^+

Tubule cell

NB cell membrane impermeable to HCO_3^-

Na^+

Carbonic anhydrase

$-50\ mV$

Na^+

LUMEN

$CO_2 \leftarrow H_2CO_3 \leftarrow H^+ + HCO_3^-$
$+ H_2O$

Basolateral membrane

K^+ Na^+

$-80\ mV$

K^+ Na^+

Carbonic anhydrase (cytosol) only

H^+

Luminal membrane

Block Na^+ channels

$-30\ mV$

K^+ Na^+ H^+

Na^+ reabsorption (stimulated by aldosterone) makes lumen more '-ve' encouraging K^+ and H^+ secretion

LUMEN

● Na^+/K^+ ATPase   ○ antiporters   ◐ synporters   ▯ channels

Diuretics are drugs that act on the kidney to increase urine flow. Most work by reducing the reabsorption of electrolytes by the tubules (top). The increased electrolyte excretion is accompanied by an increase in water excretion, necessary to maintain an osmotic balance. Diuretics are used to reduce oedema in *congestive heart failure*, some *renal diseases* and *hepatic cirrhosis*. Some diuretics, notably the thiazides, are widely used in the treatment of *hypertension*, but their long-term hypotensive action is not only related to their diuretic properties.

The **thiazides** and related compounds (top right) are safe, orally active, but relatively weak diuretics. More effective drugs are the **high ceiling** or **loop diuretics** (top left). These drugs have a very rapid onset and fairly short duration of action. They are very powerful (hence the term 'high ceiling') and can cause serious electrolyte imbalances and dehydration. **Metolazone** is a thiazide-related drug with activity between the loop and thiazide diuretics. It has a powerful synergistic

action with frusemide and the combination may be effective in resistant oedema and in patients with seriously impaired renal failure. The thiazides, and the loop diuretics, increase potassium excretion and potassium supplements may be required to prevent hypokalaemia.

Some diuretics are '**potassium sparing**' (bottom right). They are weak when used alone, but they cause potassium retention, and are often given with thiazides or loop diuretics to prevent hypokalaemia.

Carbonic anhydrase inhibitors (bottom left figure) are weak diuretics and are rarely used for their diuretic action. **Osmotic diuretics** (e.g. *mannitol*) are compounds that are filtered but not reabsorbed. They are excreted with an osmotic equivalent of water and are used in cerebral oedema, and sometimes to maintain a diuresis during surgery.

The kidney is one of the major routes of drug elimination, and impairment of renal function in old age or in renal disease can significantly decrease the elimination of drugs.

Aldosterone stimulates Na^+ reabsorption in the distal tubule and increases K^+ and H^+ secretion. It acts on cytoplasmic receptors (Chapter 33) and induces the synthesis of Na^+/K^+ ATPase in the basolateral membrane and a protein, which increases the permeability of the Na^+ channels. A more rapid increase in Na^+-channel permeability may be mediated by cell surface aldosterone receptors. Diuretics *increase* the Na^+ load in the distal tubule and, except for the potassium sparing agents, this results in an *increased K^+ secretion* (and excretion). This effect is greater if plasma aldosterone levels are high; for example if vigorous diuretic therapy has depleted the body of Na^+ stores.

Carbonic anhydrase inhibitors depress bicarbonate reabsorption in the proximal tubule by inhibiting the catalysis of CO_2 hydration and dehydration reactions. Thus, the excretion of HCO_3^-, Na^+ and H_2O is increased. The loss of HCO_3^- causes a metabolic acidosis and the effects of the drug become self-limiting as the blood bicarbonate falls. The increased Na^+ delivered to the distal nephron increases K^+ secretion. **Acetazolamide** is used in the treatment of glaucoma to reduce intraocular pressure, which it does by reducing the secretion of HCO_3^- and associated H_2O into the aqueous humour (Chapter 10). It is also used as a prophylactic agent for mountain (altitude) sickness.

THIAZIDES

Thiazides were developed from the carbonic anhydrase inhibitors. However, the diuretic activity of these drugs is not related to their effects on this enzyme. The thiazides are widely used in the treatment of mild heart failure (Chapter 18) and hypertension (Chapter 15), in which condition they have been shown to reduce the incidence of stroke. There are many thiazides but the only major difference is their duration of action. **Bendrofluazide** is widely used.

Mechanism. Thiazides act mainly on the early segments of the *distal tubule*, where they *inhibit NaCl reabsorption* by binding to the synporter responsible for the electroneutral cotransport of Na^+–Cl^-. Excretion of Cl^-, Na^+ and accompanying H_2O is increased. The increased Na^+ load in the distal tubule stimulates Na^+ exchange with K^+ and H^+, increasing their excretion and causing hypokalaemia and a metabolic alkalosis.

Adverse effects include *weakness, impotence* and occasionally *skin rashes*. Serious allergic reactions (e.g. thrombocytopenia) are rare. More common are metabolic effects:
1 **Hypokalaemia** may precipitate cardiac arrhythmias, especially in patients on digitalis. This can be prevented by giving potassium supplements if necessary, or by combined therapy with a potassium-sparing diuretic.
2 **Hyperuricaemia.** Uric acid levels in the blood are often increased because thiazides are secreted by the organic acid secretory system in the tubules and compete for uric acid secretion. This may precipitate *gout*.
3 **Glucose tolerance** may be impaired and thiazides are contraindicated in patients with non-insulin-dependent diabetes.
4 **Lipids.** Thiazides increase plasma cholesterol levels at least during the first 6 months of administration but this is of uncertain significance.

LOOP DIURETICS

Loop diuretics (usually **frusemide**) are used to reduce peripheral and pulmonary oedema in moderate and severe heart failure (Chapter 18). They are given intravenously to patients with pulmonary oedema that results from acute ventricular failure. Unlike the thiazides, loop diuretics are effective in patients with diminished renal function.

Mechanism. Loop agents have a thiazide-like action on the early distal tubule but, much more importantly, they *inhibit NaCl reabsorption* in the *thick ascending loop of Henle*. This segment has a high capacity for absorbing NaCl and so drugs which act on this site produce a diuresis that is much greater than that of other diuretics. Loop diuretics act on the luminal membrane where they inhibit the cotransport of Na^+–K^+–$2Cl^-$. (The Na^+ is actively transported out of the cells into the interstitium by a Na^+/K^+ ATPase-dependent pump in the basolateral membrane.) The specificity of the loop diuretics is due to their high local concentration in the renal tubules. However, at high doses these drugs may induce changes in the electrolyte composition of the endolymph and cause deafness.

Adverse effects. Like the thiazides, the loop agents have *hyperglycaemic, hyperuricaemic, hypotensive* and *hypokalaemic* effects. Potassium loss, as with the thiazides, is often clinically unimportant unless there are additional risk factors for arrhythmias (e.g. digoxin treatment). Overenthusiastic use of loop diuretics (high doses, intravenous administration) can cause *deafness*, which may not be reversible.

POTASSIUM-SPARING DIURETICS

These diuretics act on the aldosterone-responsive segments of the distal nephron, where K^+ homeostasis is controlled. *Aldosterone* stimulates Na^+ reabsorption, generating a negative potential in the lumen, which drives K^+ and H^+ ions into the lumen (and hence their excretion). The potassium-sparing diuretics reduce Na^+ reabsorption by either antagonizing aldosterone (**spironolactone**) or blocking Na^+ channels (**amiloride, triamterene**). This causes the electrical potential across the tubular epithelium to fall, reducing the driving force for K^+ secretion. The drugs may cause *severe hyperkalaemia*, especially in patients with renal impairment. Hyperkalaemia is also likely to occur if patients are also taking inhibitors of angiotensin converting enzyme (e.g. captopril), because these drugs reduce aldosterone secretion (and therefore K^+ excretion).

Spironolactone competitively blocks the binding of aldosterone to its cytoplasmic receptor and so increases the excretion of Na^+ (Cl^- and H_2O) and decreases the 'electrically coupled' K^+ secretion. It is a weak diuretic, because only 2% of the total Na^+ reabsorption is under aldosterone control. Some metabolites of spironolactone have been shown to be carcinogenic in rats and the drug is now only used in liver disease with ascites and Conn's syndrome (primary hyperaldosteronism).

Amiloride and **triamterene** decrease the luminal membrane Na^+ permeability in the distal nephron by combining with Na^+ channels and blocking them on a 1:1 basis. This increases Na^+ (Cl^- and H_2O) excretion and decreases K^+ excretion.

15 Drugs used in hypertension

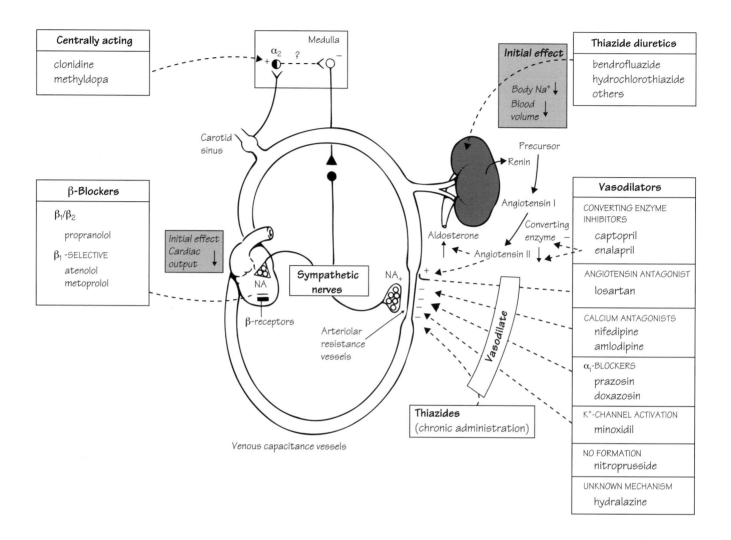

High blood pressure is associated with decreased life expectancy and increased risk of stroke, coronary heart disease and other end-organ disease (e.g. retinopathy, renal failure). The problem is that the risk is graded and so there is no obvious line between patients who should be treated and those who should not. Lowering the blood pressure of patients with a diastolic blood pressure of above 90 mmHg decreases mortality and morbidity but this could include 25% of the population. In the UK, it is generally accepted that in patients without additional risk factors, therapy is indicated if the diastolic pressure is greater than 100 mmHg and/or the systolic pressure is greater than 160 mmHg. Other risk factors for vascular disease that may be supra-additive include smoking (discourage strongly), obesity, hyperlipidaemia, diabetes and left ventricular hypertrophy. A few patients have hypertension secondary to renal or endocrine disease.

In some patients with mild hypertension, weight reduction, if appropriate, reduced alcohol consumption and moderate reduction in salt consumption may be sufficient, but usually drug treatment is required. The **β-adrenoceptor antagonists** (β-blockers, centre left) and the **thiazide diuretics** (top right) are presently the first-line drugs in the treatment of hypertension. In neither case is their mode of action clear. Several groups of drugs, by different mechanisms, reduce blood pressure by decreasing vasoconstrictor tone and hence peripheral resistance. The most important of these are the angiotensin converting enzyme (**ACE**) inhibitors (middle right), which decrease circulating angiotensin II (a vasoconstrictor), and the **calcium antagonists** (middle right), which block the entry of calcium into vascular smooth muscle cells. Other vasodilators (bottom right) have been largely superseded by the ACE inhibitors and calcium antagonists, although there is some interest in selective α_1-**adrenoceptor antagonists**, mainly because it is claimed that they have 'favourable' effects on blood lipids. **Centrally acting drugs** (top left) decrease sympathetic outflow by stimulating central α_2-adrenoceptors, but are little used currently because of their adverse effects.

Mild to moderate hypertension can often be controlled by a single drug (usually a thiazide or β-blocker), but if this fails the traditional approach is to combine two drugs (e.g. diuretic and β-blocker; diuretic and ACE inhibitor) and add a third if necessary, usually a long-acting α_1-blocker such as doxazosin.

THIAZIDE DIURETICS

The mechanism by which diuretics reduce arterial blood pressure is not known. Initially, the blood pressure falls because of a decrease in blood volume, venous return and cardiac output. Gradually, the cardiac output returns to normal but the hypotensive effect remains because the peripheral resistance has, in the meantime, decreased. Diuretics have no direct effect on vascular smooth muscle and the vasodilatation they cause seems to be associated with a small but persistent reduction in body Na^+. One possible mechanism is that a fall in smooth muscle Na^+ causes a secondary reduction in intracellular Ca^{2+} so that the muscle becomes less responsive. Thiazide diuretics may cause *hypokalaemia*, *diabetes mellitus*, *gout* and change the blood lipids in an 'atherogenic' way (see also Chapter 14). Side effects such as impotence and loss of libido were reported to be more common with thiazide usage than with β-blockers but it is now appreciated that thiazides have a flat dose–response curve and the low doses of thiazides currently used to lower blood pressure cause insignificant metabolic effects.

β-ADRENOCEPTOR ANTAGONISTS

β-Blockers initially produce a fall in blood pressure by decreasing the cardiac output. With continued treatment, the cardiac output returns to normal but the blood pressure remains low, because, by an unknown mechanism, the peripheral vascular resistance is 'reset' at a lower level (individual drugs are discussed in Chapter 9). Disadvantages of β-blockade are the common adverse effects, such as cold hands and fatigue, and the less common, but serious, adverse effects, such as the *provocation of asthma*, *heart failure* or *conductance block*. β-Blockers also tend to raise serum triglyceride and decrease high density lipoprotein–cholesterol levels. All the β-blockers lower blood pressure but at least some of the side effects can be reduced by using cardioselective hydrophilic drugs (i.e. those without liver metabolism or brain penetration) such as atenolol.

VASODILATOR DRUGS

ACE inhibitors. Angiotensin II is a powerful circulating vasoconstrictor and inhibition of its synthesis in hypertensive subjects results in a fall in peripheral resistance and a lowering of blood pressure. ACE inhibitors do not impair cardiovascular reflexes and are devoid of many of the adverse effects of the diuretics and β-blockers. A comon unwanted effect of ACE inhibitors is a dry cough that may be caused by increased bradykinin (ACE also metabolizes bradykinin). Rare but serious adverse effects of ACE inhibitors include angio-oedema, proteinuria and neutropenia. The first dose may cause a very steep fall in blood pressure, e.g. in patients on diuretics (because they are Na^+ depleted). ACE inhibitors may cause renal failure in patients with bilateral renal artery stenosis, because in this condition angiotensin II is apparently required to constrict postglomerular arterioles and maintain adequate glomerular filtration. Inhibition of angiotensin II formation reduces, but does not seriously impair, aldosterone secretion, and excessive K^+ retention only occurs in patients taking potassium supplements or potassium-sparing diuretics (aldosterone increases Na^+ reabsorption and K^+ excretion, Chapter 14).

Angiotensin receptor antagonist. Losartan is a new drug that lowers the blood pressure by blocking angiotensin (AT_1) receptors. It does not cause cough, perhaps because it does not prevent bradykinin degradtion.

Calcium antagonists (see also Chapters 16 & 17). The tone of vascular smooth muscle is determined by the cytosolic Ca^{2+} concentration. This is increased by α_1-adrenoceptor activation (resulting from sympathetic tone) which triggers Ca^{2+} release from the sarcoplasmic reticulum via the second-messenger inositol trisphosphate (Chapter 1). There also seem to be receptor-operated cation channels, about which little is known. Nevertheless, they are important because the entry of cations through them depolarizes the cell, opening voltage-dependent (L-type) Ca^{2+} channels which causes additional Ca^{2+} to enter the cell. The calcium antagonists (e.g. **nifedipine**, **amlodipine**) bind to the L-type channels and by blocking the entry of Ca^{2+} into the cell they cause relaxation of the arteriolar smooth muscle. This reduces the peripheral resistance and results in a fall in blood pressure. The efficacy of calcium antagonists is similar to that of the thiazides and β-blockers. Their most common side effects are due to excessive vasodilatation and include dizziness, hypotension, flushing and ankle oedema.

α-Adrenoceptor antagonists. Prazosin and the longer acting **doxazosin** cause vasodilatation by selectively blocking vascular α_1-adrenoceptors. Unlike non-selective α-blockers, these drugs are not likely to cause tachycardia, but they may cause postural hypotension. Severe hypotension may occur after the first dose.

Hydralazine is used in combination with a β-blocker and diuretic. Side effects include reflex tachycardia, which may provoke angina, headaches and fluid retention (due to secondary hyperaldosteronism). In slow acetylators in particular, hydralazine may induce a *lupus syndrome* resulting in fever, arthralgia, malaise and hepatitis.

Minoxidil (active metabolite, minoxidil sulphate) is a potent vasodilator which causes severe fluid retention and oedema. However, when given with a β-blocker and loop diuretic, it is effective in severe hypertension resistant to other drug combinations. Minoxidil sulphate opens ATP-sensitive K^+ channels in vascular smooth muscle cells, causing hyperpolarization and relaxation. These K^+ channels are normally kept closed by intracellular ATP, which is apparently antagonized by minoxidil sulphate (cf. oral antidiabetic drugs, Chapter 36).

CENTRALLY ACTING DRUGS

Methyldopa is converted in adrenergic nerve endings to the false transmitter, α-methylnoradrenaline, which stimulates α_2 receptors in the medulla and reduces sympathetic outflow. Drowsiness is common and in 20% of patients it causes a positive antiglobulin (Coombs') test and, rarely, haemolytic anaemia (Chapter 45). **Clonidine** causes rebound hypertension if the drug is suddenly withdrawn.

ACUTE SEVERE HYPERTENSION

In hypertensive crisis drugs may be given by intravenous infusion (e.g. **hydralazine** in hypertension associated with eclampsia of pregnancy; **nitroprusside** in malignant hypertension with encephalopathy). However, intravenous drugs are rarely necessary, and the trend is to use oral agents whenever possible. Nitroprusside decomposes in the blood to release nitric oxide (NO), an unstable compound that causes vasodilatation (see Chapter 16 for mechanism).

16 Drugs used in angina

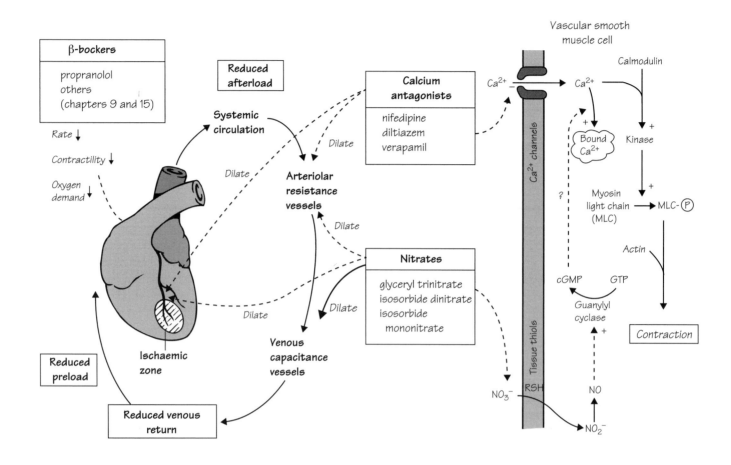

The coronary arteries supply blood to the heart. With increasing age atheromatous plaques progressively narrow the arteries, and the obstruction to blood flow may eventually become so severe that when exercise increases the oxygen consumption of the heart, not enough blood can pass through the arteries to supply it. The ischaemic muscle then produces the characteristic symptoms of **angina pectoris**, probably because waste products released during muscle contraction accumulate in the poorly perfused tissue.

The basic aim of drug treatment in angina is to reduce the work of the heart and hence its oxygen demand. The **nitrates** (lower middle) are the first-line drugs. Their main effect is to cause peripheral vasodilatation, especially in the veins, by an action on the vascular smooth muscle that involves the formation of nitric oxide (NO) and an increase in intracellular cGMP (right figure). The resulting pooling of blood in the capacitance vessels (veins) reduces venous return and the ventricular volume is decreased. Reduction in the distension of the heart wall decreases oxygen demand and the pain is quickly relieved. **Glyceryl trinitrate** given sublingually to avoid first-pass metabolism is used to treat acute anginal attacks. If this is ineffective then combined therapy is required in which β-**adrenoceptor blockers** (top left) or **calcium antagonists** (middle top) are taken in addition to glyceryl trinitrate, which is retained for acute attacks.

β-**Adrenoceptor blockers** depress myocardial contractility and reduce the heart rate. In addition to these effects, which reduce the oxygen demand, β-blockers may also increase the perfusion of the ischaemic area, because the decrease in heart rate increases the duration of diastole and hence the time available for coronary blood flow.

β-Blockers are the standard drugs used in angina, but they have many side effects and contraindications (Chapter 15). If β-blockers cannot be used, e.g. in patients with asthma, then a calcium antagonist can be used as an adjunct to short-acting nitrates. Calcium antagonists have actions on the heart, but they relieve angina mainly by causing peripheral arteriolar dilatation and afterload reduction. They are especially useful if there is some degree of coronary artery spasm. Recent evidence suggests that short-acting calcium antagonists (e.g. nifedipine and diltiazem) may increase mortality in patients with angina (and perhaps hypertension). Long-acting preparations of these drugs are now available, but the safest choice seems to be verapamil or amlodipine, which can be given once daily.

In **unstable angina**, antiplatelet therapy with **aspirin** reduces the risk of myocardial infarction. It also improves the survival of patients with acute myocardial infarction and reduces the incidence of a second infarction (Chapter 19).

Angina pectoris is a description of a typical set of symptoms related to myocardial ischaemia and usually due to underlying atheromatous narrowing of the coronary arteries. These symptoms include a feeling of tightness in the chest, usually retrosternal and often radiating to the arms, precipitated by exercise and relieved by rest and nitrates.

Stable and unstable angina. In 'stable' angina there is little change in the pain or the frequency of the attacks. When, however, the symptoms are of sudden or recent onset, or are progressing in severity or frequency, occurring at lesser levels of exertion or at rest, the term 'unstable angina' may be applied. Unstable angina has a different pathology and probably results from fissuring of an atheromatous plaque with subsequent platelet aggregation. In these patients, antiplatelet treatment with aspirin reduces the probability of myocardial infarction by approximately 50%.

NITRATES

Short-acting nitrates. Glyceryl trinitrate (sublingual tablet or spray) acts for about 30 minutes. It is more useful in preventing attacks than in stopping them once they have begun. Patches containing glycerol trinitrate (transdermal administration) have a long duration of action (up to 24 hours).

Long-acting nitrates are more stable and may be effective for several hours, depending on the drug and preparation used (sublingual, oral, oral sustained-release). **Isosorbide dinitrate** is widely used, but it is rapidly metabolized by the liver. The use of **isosorbide mononitrate**, which is the main active metabolite of the dinitrate, avoids the variable absorption and unpredictable first-pass metabolism of the dinitrate. The prophylactic value of long-acting nitrates is uncertain, but they are a rational choice for the acute treatment of unstable angina.

Adverse effects. The arterial dilatation produced by the nitrates causes headaches, which frequently limit the dose. More serious side effects are hypotension and fainting. Reflex tachycardia often occurs but this is prevented by combined therapy with β-blockers. Prolonged high dosage may cause methaemoglobinaemia due to oxidation of haemoglobin.

Mechanism of action. Metabolism of the drugs first releases nitrite ions (NO_2^-), a process that requires tissue thiols. Within the cell, NO_2^- is converted to nitric oxide (NO) which then activates guanylyl cyclase, causing an increase in the intracellular concentration of guanosine $3',5'$-monophosphate (cGMP) in the vascular smooth muscle cells. Precisely how the cGMP causes relaxation is not clear, but it eventually results in the dephosphorylation of the myosin light chain (MLC), possibly by decreasing the concentration of free Ca^{2+} ions in the cytosol. (Phosphorylation of MLC initiates the interaction of myosin with actin and muscle contraction.)

Tolerance may occur to nitrates. For example, chronic pentaerythritol tetranitrate has been shown to produce tolerance to sublingual glyceryl trinitrate, and moderate doses of oral isosorbide dinitrate four times a day produce tolerance with loss of the anti-anginal effect. However, twice daily dosing of isosorbide dinitrate at 0800 and 1300 hours does not produce tolerance, presumably because the overnight rest allows tissue sensitivity to return by the next day. Tolerance to nitrates is poorly understood but depletion of sulphydryl group donors may be involved, since tolerance to nitrates *in vitro* can sometimes be reversed by *N*-acetylcysteine.

β-ADRENOCEPTOR ANTAGONISTS

β-Blockers are used for prophylaxis of angina. The choice of drug may be important. *Intrinsic activity might be* a *disadvantage* in angina, and the cardioselective β-blockers such as **atenolol** and **metoprolol** are probably the drugs of choice. All β-blockers must be avoided in asthmatics as they may precipitate bronchospasm. The *adverse effects* and contraindications of β-blockers should be reviewed (Chapters 9 and 15).

CALCIUM ANTAGONISTS

These drugs are widely used in the treatment of angina and have fewer serious side effects than β-blockers. Calcium antagonists block L-type voltage-sensitive calcium channels in arterial smooth muscle, causing relaxation and vasodilatation (Chapter 15). Preload is not significantly affected. Calcium channels in the myocardium and conducting tissues of the heart are also affected by calcium antagonists, which produce a negative inotropic effect by reducing calcium influx during the plateau phase of the action potential. However, the dihydropyridines (e.g. **nifedipine, amlodipine**) have relatively little effect on the heart because at clinically used doses, vasodilatation results in a reflex increase in sympathetic tone that causes a mild tachycardia and counteracts the mild negative inotropic effect. **Amlodipine**, which has a long duration of action, produces less tachycardia than nifedipine. **Verapamil** and, to a lesser extent, **diltiazem** depress the sinus node, causing a mild resting bradycardia. Conduction in the atrioventricular node is slowed and because the effect of verapamil (unlike nifedipine) is frequency dependent, it effectively slows the ventricular rate in atrial arrhythmias (Chapter 17). The negative inotropic effects of verapamil and diltiazem are partially offset by the reflex increase in adrenergic tone and the decrease in afterload. Verapamil is not used in angina because it may cause heart failure or AV block. Diltiazem has actions intermediate between those of verapamil and nifedipine and is popular in the treatment of angina because it does not cause tachycardia.

Tobacco smoking. Smoking is prothrombotic and atherogenic, it reduces coronary blood flow and the nicotine-induced rise in heart rate and blood pressure increases the oxygen demand of the heart. In addition, the formation of carboxyhaemoglobin reduces the oxygen-carrying capacity of the blood. Some patients improve remarkably on giving up smoking.

Coronary artery bypass or **percutaneous transarterial coronary angioplasty (PTCA)** may be indicated in patients not responding to drugs. In bypass operations, a segment of saphenous vein or internal mammary artery is inserted between the aorta and a point beyond the stenosis of the affected coronary artery. Angina is relieved or improved in 90% of patients, but returns in 50% within 7 years. Mortality is decreased in some pathological conditions (e.g. left main coronary artery disease). In PTCA a balloon catheter is used to split and compress the atheromatous plaque.

17 Anti-arrhythmic drugs

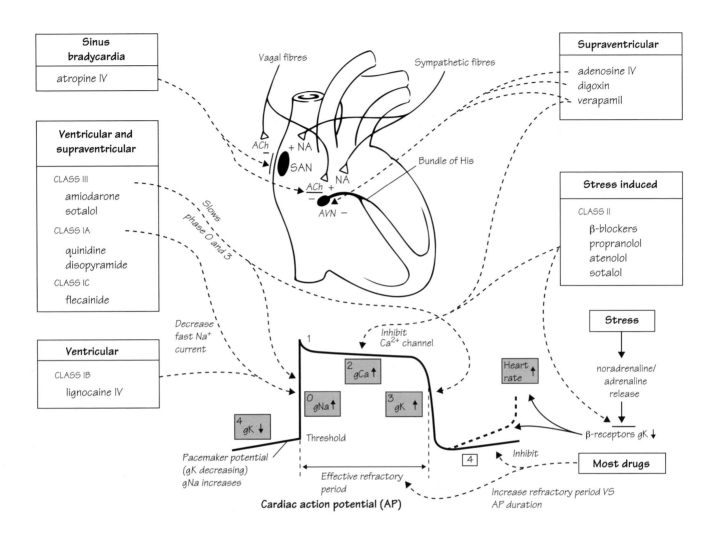

The rhythm of the heart is normally determined by **pacemaker** cells in the sinoatrial node (SAN, top), but it can be disturbed in a variety of ways, producing anything from occasional discomfort to the symptoms of heart failure or even sudden death. Arrhythmias can occur in the apparently healthy heart, but serious ones (i.e. ventricular tachycardias) are usually associated with heart disease (e.g. myocardial infarction). The rhythm of the heart is affected by both **acetylcholine** (ACh) and **noradrenaline** (NA), released from parasympathetic and sympathetic nerves, respectively (upper figure).

Supraventricular arrhythmias arise in the atrial myocardium or atrioventricular node (AVN), whilst ventricular arrhythmias originate in the ventricles. Arrhythmias may be caused by an **ectopic focus**, which starts firing at a higher rate than the normal pacemaker (SAN). More commonly a **re-entry** mechanism is involved, where action potentials, delayed for some pathological reason, re-invade nearby muscle fibres which, being no longer refractory, again depolarize, establishing a loop of depolarization (circus movement).

Many anti-arrhythmic drugs have local anaesthetic activity (i.e. block voltage-dependent Na⁺ channels) or are calcium antagonists. These actions decrease the automaticity of pacemaker cells and increase the effective refractory period of atrial, ventricular and Purkinje fibres.

Anti-arrhythmic agents can be classified into:

1 those which are effective in **supraventricular arrhythmias** (top right);

2 those effective in **ventricular arrhythmias** (bottom left); and

3 those effective on **both types** (middle left).

Arrhythmias associated with stress conditions in which there is an increase in adrenergic activity (emotion, excitement, thyrotoxicosis, myocardial infarction) may be treated with β-blockers (bottom right). An arrhythmia common after acute myocardial infarction is sinus bradycardia, which can be treated with intravenous atropine if the cardiac output is lowered (top left). Anti-arrhythmics have also been classified on the basis of their electrophysiological effects on Purkinje fibres (roman numerals). The effects of anti-arrhythmic agents on the **cardiac action potential** are shown in the lower figure, but it is not usually known how these actions relate to the drugs' therapeutic effects. Many anti-arrhythmic drugs can actually induce lethal arrhythmias, especially in patients with ischaemic heart disease. Except for β-blockers in myocardial infarction there is no evidence that anti-arrhythmic drugs reduce mortality in any condition.

CARDIAC ACTION POTENTIAL

Cardiac cells have two depolarizing currents, a fast Na^+ current and a slower Ca^{2+} current. In the SAN and AVN there is only a Ca^{2+} current and because pure 'Ca^{2+} spikes' conduct very slowly, there is a delay between atrial and ventricular contraction. The long refractory period of cardiac fibres normally protects them from re-excitation during a heart beat.

PACEMAKER CELLS

In the SAN and AVN, pacemaker cells possess a K^+ conductance that gradually decreases, resulting in a depolarization drift. When the depolarization reaches threshold, an action potential is initiated. The slope of the pacemaker potentials in the SAN is greater than in the AVN and so the SAN normally determines the heart rate (sinus rhythm). The pacemaker and conducting cells receive autonomic innervation.

Acetylcholine. Vagal fibres release acetylcholine onto M_2-muscarinic receptors, the activation of which increases the K^+ conductance (gK) and decreases the slope of the pacemaker potential. Thus, the threshold for firing is reached later and the heart beat slows. Conductance in the bundle of His is also slowed.

Noradrenaline. Sympathetic fibres release noradrenaline onto β_1-receptors in the pacemaker tissues and myocardium. Noradrenaline decreases gK, so threshold is reached earlier and the heart rate increases (positive chronotropic effect). Noradrenaline also increases the force of contraction by increasing the influx of calcium during the plateau phase (positive inotropic effect).

DRUGS USED IN SUPRAVENTRICULAR ARRHYTHMIAS

Digoxin stimulates vagal activity (Chapter 18), causing the release of ACh which slows conduction and prolongs the refractory period in the AVN and bundle of His. Oral administration of digoxin is used in atrial fibrillation, where the atria beat at such high rates that the ventricles can only follow irregularly. By delaying AV conductance, digoxin increases the degree of block and slows and strengthens the ventricular beat.

Adenosine stimulates A_1-adenosine receptors and opens ACh-sensitive K^+ channels. This hyperpolarizes the cell membrane in the AVN and by inhibiting the calcium channels slows conduction in the AVN. Adenosine is rapidly inactivated ($t_{1/2;} = 8$–10 seconds) and so side effects (e.g. dyspnoea, bronchospasm) are short-lived. Intravenous adenosine is used to terminate paroxysmal supraventricular tachycardia.

Verapamil acts by blocking L-type calcium channels (**class IV agents**) (see also Chapters 15 & 16) and has particularly powerful effects on the AVN where conduction is entirely dependent on calcium spikes. It also inhibits the influx of Ca^{2+} during the plateau phase of the action potential and therefore has a negative ionotropic action. Adenosine has largely replaced intravenous verapamil for the treatment of supraventricular tachycardias because it is safer, especially if the patient really has a ventricular tachycardia, in which case the negative ionotropic effect of verapamil may be disastrous. Oral verapamil is still used in the prophylaxis of supraventricular tachycardia. Verapamil should not be used with β-blockers or quinidine because of cumulative negative ionotropic effects.

DRUGS EFFECTIVE IN SUPRAVENTRICULAR AND VENTRICULAR ARRHYTHMIAS

Class III agents act by slowing repolarization (phase 3) and prolonging the action potential and refractory period in all cardiac tissues. **Amiodarone** has blocking actions on several channels (e.g. K^+ and inactivated Na^+ channels) and β-adrenoceptors. Amiodarone is often effective when other drugs have failed but its use is restricted to patients in whom other drugs are ineffective because it may cause serious adverse effects including photosensitivity, thyroid disorders, neuropathy and pulmonary alveolitis. **Sotalol** has class III actions as well as class II (β-blocking) actions. It lacks the side effects of amiodarone but has the usual side effects of β-blockers.

Class IA agents act by blocking (open) voltage-dependent Na^+ channels. They slow phase 0 and lengthen the effective refractory period. Class IA agents produce a frequency (use)-dependent block. During diastole when the Na^+ channels are closed class IA agents dissociate relatively slowly, so if the frequency is high drug is still bound to the channel, which therefore cannot contribute to the action potential.

Disopyramide is mainly used orally to prevent recurrent ventricular arrhythmias. Disopyramide has a negative inotropic action and may cause hypotension (especially intravenously) and aggravate cardiac failure. Other side effects include nausea, vomiting and marked anticholinergic effects, which may limit its use in men (urinary retention).

Quinidine is effective in the treatment of both supraventricular and ventricular arrhythmias, but its use is limited by potentially dangerous cardiac and frequent non-cardiac side effects. Side effects include anticholinergic effects, nausea, vomiting, diarrhoea and arrhythmias.

DRUGS USED IN VENTRICULAR ARRHYTHMIAS

Class IB agents block (inactivated) voltage-dependent Na^+ channels. **Lignocaine** given intravenously is used in the treatment of ventricular arrhythmias, usually after an acute myocardial infarction. In contrast to class IA agents, which block open Na^+ channels, lignocaine blocks mainly inactivated Na^+ channels. In normal cardiac tissue, lignocaine has little effect because it dissociates rapidly from the Na^+ channels, which therefore recover during diastole. However, in ischaemic areas, where anoxia causes depolarization and arrhythmogenic activity, many Na^+ channels are inactivated and therefore susceptible to lignocaine.

ALTERNATIVES TO DRUGS

Pacemakers are required for complete heart block, and are sometimes used in tachyarrhythmias. When the left atrial size is normal, direct current shock causes reversion to sinus rhythm in most patients with atrial fibrillation, but about 60% relapse within 1 year, despite maintenance treatment with disopyramide. Surgical ablation of the ectopic focus or bundle of His is a successful method of controlling supraventricular arrhythmias. A much safer method is ablation of the focus or bundle via electrodes on an intracardiac catheter (endocavity ablation). Since AV block is produced, a permanent pacemaker is required.

18 Drugs used in heart failure

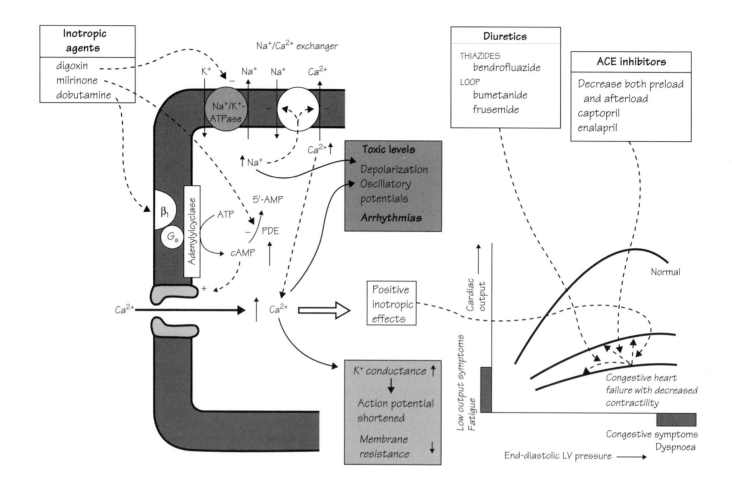

Heart failure exists when the cardiac output is insufficient to adequately perfuse the tissues. This leads to a variety of symptoms, e.g. fatigue, oedema and breathlessness. *Congestive heart failure* is usually taken to mean combined right and left heart failure, producing both pulmonary congestion and peripheral oedema. Common causes of heart failure include hypertension and coronary heart disease. The low cardiac output in heart failure results in increased sympathetic nervous activity, which stimulates the rate and force of the heart beat and maintains the blood pressure by increasing the vascular resistance. The resulting increase in afterload further depresses cardiac output. Reduced renal blood flow results in *renin secretion* and increased plasma *angiotensin* and *aldosterone* levels. Sodium and water retention increase the blood volume, increasing the preload and the likelihood of oedema formation.

Treatment of heart failure usually starts with **diuretics** (top centre) (Chapter 14), which increase the excretion of sodium and water and, by reducing the circulatory volume, decrease the preload and oedema (curved arrow, right figure). In mild heart failure a thiazide (e.g. bendrofluazide) may be sufficient but in more severe cases a loop diuretic is used. If the response to diuretics is not adequate, then a vasodilator is added, usually an **angiotensin converting enzyme (ACE) inhibitor** (top right). ACE inhibitors (e.g. **captopril**) reduce the load on the heart (diagonal arrow, right figure) and clinical trials have shown that they decrease symptoms and prolong life in congestive heart failure. If heart failure is so severe that a combination of diuretic and ACE inhibitor fails to provide an adequate response, then an **inotropic drug** (top left) may be added.

Inotropic drugs all increase the force of cardiac muscle contraction (vertical arrow, right figure) by increasing the rise in cytosolic calcium that occurs with each action potential (left figure). Thus, both β-adrenoceptor agonists (e.g. **dobutamine**) and phosphodiesterase inhibitors (e.g. **milrinone**) increase the influx of Ca^{2+} via an increase in cAMP levels (left figure), whilst **digoxin** increases intracellular calcium indirectly, by inhibiting membrane Na^+/K^+ ATPase (⬤). Inotropic drugs all tend to cause arrhythmias because excessive cytosolic calcium can trigger arrhythmogenic membrane currents. **Digoxin** is the main inotropic drug, but in acute severe heart failure where there is life-threatening hypoperfusion of the brain and kidneys (cardiogenic shock), dobutamine is given often together with dopamine by intravenous infusion.

VASODILATOR DRUGS

Venous dilatation reduces the filling pressure (preload) and arteriolar dilatation lowers the resistance against which the heart has to pump (the afterload). The reduction in vascular tone decreases the work and oxygen demand of the failing heart. ACE inhibitors (e.g. **captopril**, **enalapril**) (see also Chapter 15) are the most appropriate vasodilators in heart failure, because they lower both the arterial and venous resistance by preventing the increase in (vasoconstrictor) angiotensin II that is often present in heart failure. The cardiac output increases and because the renovascular resistance falls, there is an increase in renal blood flow. This latter effect, together with reduced aldosterone release (angiotensin II is a stimulus for aldosterone release), increases Na^+ and H_2O excretion, contracting the blood volume and reducing venous return to the heart. Other vasodilators are now only used in patients who cannot tolerate ACE inhibitors.

INOTROPIC DRUGS

Digoxin is a glycoside extracted from foxglove leaves, *Digitalis* sp. It consists of a steroid ring structure (aglycone), which possesses the pharmacological activity, combined with sugar molecules (digitoxose) that enhance binding.

Mechanical effects and therapeutic benefit. Digoxin increases the force of cardiac contraction in the failing heart and reduces its oxygen consumption. This action is responsible for the therapeutic benefit of digitalis in heart failure. This benefit has often been doubted in patients with chronic heart failure in sinus rhythm, but recent clinical trials have shown that digoxin can reduce the symptoms of heart failure in patients who are already receiving diuretics. Digoxin is particularly indicated in heart failure due to atrial fibrillation (Chapter 17).

Mechanism of action. Digoxin inhibits membrane Na^+/K^+ ATPase (●), which is responsible for Na^+/K^+ exchange across the muscle cell membrane. This increases intracellular Na^+ and produces a secondary increase in intracellular Ca^{2+} which increases the force of myocardial contraction. The increase in intracellular Ca^{2+} occurs because the decreased Na^+ gradient across the membrane reduces the extrusion of Ca^{2+} by the Na^+/Ca^{2+} exchanger (○) that occurs during diastole.

Digoxin and K^+ ions compete for a 'receptor' (Na^+/K^+ ATPase) on the outside of the muscle cell membrane, so the effects of digoxin may be *dangerously increased in hypokalaemia*, produced, for example, by diuretics.

Electrical effects. These are due to a complicated mixture of direct and indirect actions.

Direct effects (bottom, ■). At non-toxic concentrations: (i) the cardiac action potential is shortened and the membrane resistance is lowered, probably because of the increased intracellular Ca^{2+}, which is known to increase the potassium conductance; (ii) shortening of the action potential shortens the atrial and ventricular refractory period; and (iii) toxic concentrations (top, ■) cause depolarization (due to Na^+ pump inhibition), and oscillatory depolarizing afterpotentials appear after normal action potentials (caused by increased intracellular Ca^{2+}). If the afterpotential reaches threshold an action potential is gen-

erated, causing an 'ectopic beat'. With increasing toxicity the ectopic beat itself elicits further beats, causing a self-sustaining arrhythmia (ventricular tachycardia), which may progress to ventricular fibrillation.

Indirect effects. Digoxin increases central vagal activity and facilitates muscarinic transmission in the heart. This: (i) slows the heart rate; (ii) slows atrioventricular conductance; and (iii) prolongs the refractory period of the atrioventricular node and bundle of His. *Use is made of this effect in atrial fibrillation* (Chapter 17), but at toxic levels heart block occurs.

Effects on other organs. Digoxin affects all excitable tissues, its cardioselectivity resulting from a greater dependence of myocardial function on the rate of sodium extrusion. The most common extracardiac action is on the gut, and digoxin may cause anorexia, nausea, vomiting or diarrhoea. These effects are partly due to actions on the smooth muscle of the gut and partly a result of central vagal and chemoreceptor trigger zone stimulation. Less common effects include confusion or even psychosis.

Toxicity. Digoxin toxicity is *quite common*. According to its severity, treatment may require withdrawal of the drug, potassium supplements, anti-arrhythmic drugs (phenytoin or lignocaine) or, in very severe intoxication, digoxin-specific antibody fragments (Fab).

SYMPATHOMIMETIC AGENTS

These activate cardiac β_1-receptors and stimulate adenylyl cyclase, an effect mediated by a G-protein called G_s (left). The resulting rise in cAMP activates cAMP-dependent protein kinase, which leads to phosphorylation of the L-type Ca^{2+} channels and an increase in the probability of their opening. This increases the influx of Ca^{2+} and hence the force of myocardial contraction. In general, they are little used in heart failure because they are arrhythmogenic and also increase the heart rate and oxygen consumption. This increases ischaemia and infarct size in myocardial infarction.

Dobutamine is given by intravenous infusion in *acute severe heart failure*. It stimulates β_1-adrenoceptors in the heart and increases contractility with little effect on rate.

Dopamine given by intravenous infusion also stimulates cardiac β_1-adrenoceptors. At lower doses, it increases renal perfusion by stimulating dopamine receptors in the renal vasculature. Dobutamine and low doses of dopamine are often given together in cardiogenic shock.

PHOSPHODIESTERASE INHIBITORS

Milrinone inhibits phosphodiesterase III (PDE, left figure) in the myocardial cells, causing a rise in intracellular cAMP and consequently an increase in Ca^{2+} influx. In addition to increasing myocardial contractility, milrinone is a vasodilator. It is given by intravenous infusion in severe congestive heart failure unresponsive to other therapy. There is no evidence that milrinone (or other PDE inhibitors) improves survival and it is rarely used. Chronic administration of milrinone in congestive heart failure is associated with increased mortality.

19 Drugs used to affect blood coagulation

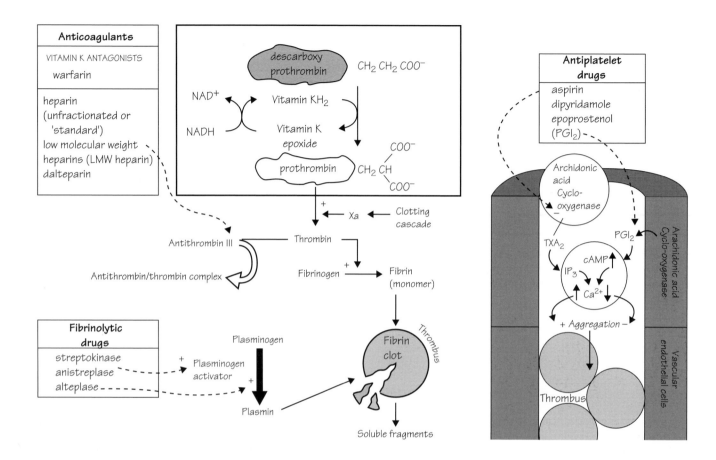

The centre of the figure shows the final stages of the cascade sequence involved in clot (thrombus) formation. In the slower moving venous side of the circulation, the thrombus (⬤) consists of a fibrin web enmeshed with platelets and red blood cells. **Anticoagulant drugs** (top left), particularly heparin and warfarin, are widely used in the prevention and treatment of *venous thrombosis* and *embolism* (e.g. deep vein thrombosis, prevention of postoperative thrombosis, atrial fibrillation, patients with artificial heart valves). The main adverse effect of anticoagulants is **haemorrhage**.

Heparin is short acting and must be given by injection. Its anticoagulant effect requires the presence of *antithrombin III*, a protease inhibitor in the blood that forms a 1 : 1 complex with thrombin (⟹). Heparin increases the *rate* of complex formation 1000-fold, causing the almost instantaneous inactivation of thrombin. The heparin–antithrombin III complex also inhibits factor Xa and some other factors. Low molecular weight (LMW) heparin–antithrombin complex inhibits only factor Xa. Heparin acts both *in vitro* and *in vivo*.

Warfarin is active orally. It is a coumarin derivative with a structure similar to that of vitamin K. Warfarin blocks vitamin K-dependent γ-carboxylation of glutamate residues (top, shaded), resulting in the production of modified factors VII, IX, X and prothrombin. These are inactive in promoting coagulation because the γ-carboxylation confers Ca^{2+}-binding properties that are essential for the proteins to assemble into an efficient catalytic complex. The oral anticoagulants are only active *in vivo* and take at least 36–48 hours for the anticoagulant effect to develop. Thus, if an immediate effect is required heparin must be given in addition.

Anticoagulants are less useful in preventing *arterial thrombosis*, because in faster-flowing vessels thrombi are composed mainly of platelets with little fibrin. **Antiplatelet drugs** (right) may inhibit platelet aggregation and arterial thrombosis. **Aspirin** is the only drug for which there is convincing evidence of antiplatelet activity. It has been shown to be beneficial in ischaemic heart disease and especially in stroke prevention. Aspirin is thought to act by inhibiting the synthesis of platelet thromboxane-A_2 (TXA_2) (right figure), which is the major eicosanoid in platelets and a powerful inducer of aggregation.

Fibrinolytic drugs (bottom left) are administered intravenously. They are agents that can rapidly lyse thrombi by activating plasminogen to form plasmin (⬇), a proteolytic enzyme that degrades fibrin and so dissolves thrombi. Thrombolytic drugs, especially streptokinase, are extensively used together with oral aspirin in the treatment of myocardial infarction, and all have been shown to decrease mortality. The beneficial effects are greatest if the drugs are given within 3 hours of myocardial infarction, with progressively less benefit over 24 hours. Rapid administration of a thrombolytic agent after infarction is more important than the choice of agent.

Thrombus is an unwanted clot inside a blood vessel. Thrombosis is particulary likely to occur where the blood flow is sluggish, because this allows activated clotting factors to accumulate instead of being washed away. A common problem is postoperative thrombosis in the leg veins. Sometimes bits of thrombus break off (emboli) and are carried to distant sites, which may be severely damaged, e.g. pulmonary embolism. In atrial fibrillation the loss of atrial contraction predisposes to stasis of blood and encourages thrombus formation. These may detach and cause cerebral embolism (stroke).

ANTICOAGULANTS

Heparin is a naturally occurring, highly acidic glycosaminoglycan of varying molecular weight (5000–15 000). Subcutaneous injections or continuous intravenous infusions of heparin reduce the incidence of deep venous thrombosis in patients undergoing general surgery and those recovering from stroke and myocardial infarction.

The main side effect of heparin is bleeding. This can usually be controlled by stopping the drug administration, since it has a short duration of action (4–6 hours). If necessary, heparin can be neutralized by the intravenous injection of protamine, a basic peptide that combines with the acidic heparin. Heparin occasionally causes allergic reactions and thrombocytopenia.

LMW heparins have a longer half-life than standard heparin and a single dose by subcutaneous injection is as effective as intravenous heparin. They are used increasingly in place of heparin.

VITAMIN K ANTAGONISTS

Warfarin is well absorbed after oral administration, but the onset of its full anticoagulant effect is delayed for 1–3 days, while the inactive coagulation factors induced by the drug gradually replace those originally present. Warfarin has a long half-life (about 40 hours) and it can take up to 5 days for the prothrombin time to return to normal after stopping treatment. It is metabolized by the liver to inactive 7-hydroxywarfarin. Drugs that induce hepatic microsomal enzymes (e.g. *barbiturates*, *carbamazepine*) antagonize the anticoagulant action of warfarin, and haemorrhage may occur if they are withdrawn. Drugs that inhibit hepatic enzymes decrease the catabolism of warfarin and potentiate its action (e.g. *cimetidine*, *ethanol*, *metronidazole*). Warfarin can be reversed by giving a concentrate of clotting factors (or fresh frozen plasma which contains clotting factors); this is the treatment of choice for rapid reversal. In severe overdosage, vitamin K (phytomenadione) can be given by intravenous injection but takes 6–12 hours to act.

ANTIPLATELET DRUGS

Aspirin reduces the risk of myocardial infarction in patients with unstable angina and increases survival in patients who have had acute myocardial infarction. It also reduces the risk of stroke in patients with transient ischaemic attacks. The beneficial effects of aspirin in thromboembolic disease are thought to be due to the inhibition of platelet TXA_2 synthesis. Thromboxane-A_2 is a powerful inducer of platelet aggregation. It acts on cell surface receptors and activates phospholipase C, causing the formation of inositol trisphosphate ($InsP_3$) and consequently a rise in intracellular calcium, which triggers aggregation. The endothelial cells of the vascular wall produce a prostaglandin, PGI_2 (prostacyclin), which may be the physiological antagonist of TXA_2. PGI_2 stimulates different receptors on the platelet and activates adenylyl cyclase. The resulting increase in cAMP is associated with a decrease in intracellular calcium and inhibition of platelet aggregation. Aspirin prevents TXA_2 formation by irreversibly inhibiting cyclo-oxygenase (Chapter 32). Platelets cannot synthesize new enzyme, but the vascular endothelial cells can, and aspirin ($320\,mg\,day^{-1}$) given on alternate days produces a selective inhibition of cyclo-oxygenase over much of the dose interval. Thus, the balance of the anti-aggregatory effects of PGI_2 and the pro-aggregatory effects of TXA_2 is shifted in a beneficial direction. **Dipyridamole** is used with warfarin to prevent thrombosis formation on prosthetic heart valves. The mechanism of action of dipyridamole is unknown and it is of doubtful efficacy.

FIBRINOLYTIC DRUGS (THROMBOLYTICS)

Fibrinolytic drugs (mainly **streptokinase** but increasingly tissue plasminogen activator (**tPA**) in the UK) are used extensively in myocardial infarction to lyse the thrombi that block coronary arteries. They are administered by intravenous infusion and probably cause reperfusion in about 50% of arteries, if given within 3 hours. *The beneficial effects of aspirin in myocardial infarction are additive to those of thrombolytics.* The main side effects of thrombolytics are nausea, vomiting, bleeding and, except for alteplase, allergic reactions. Bleeding is usually restricted to the injection site but occasionally stroke occurs. **Streptokinase** is not an enzyme, it binds to circulating plasminogen to form an activator complex which converts further plasminogen to plasmin. Because there is a large excess of plasmin inhibitors in the blood, which can neutralize circulating plasmin, bleeding is not usually a problem. Within the thrombus the concentration of plasmin inhibitors is low, and so streptokinase has some selectivity for clots.

Alteplase is human tPA produced by recombinant DNA technology. Alteplase does not cause allergic reactions and can be used in patients when recent streptococcal infections or recent use of streptokinase contraindicates the use of streptokinase (i.e. patients at some risk of anaphylaxis). In contrast to streptokinase, coadministration of heparin with alteplase produces added benefit but increases the risk of stroke. Alteplase is widely used in the USA and is particularly effective if given early.

Anistreplase is a complex of streptokinase and human plasminogen made inactive by an anisoyl group at the catalytic centre. In the blood, the anisoyl group is slowly lost to give active plasminogen–streptokinase. This lengthens the duration of action to 4–6 hours and allows it to be given as a single intravenous injection. Because it contains streptokinase, allergic reactions may occur.

20 Lipid-lowering drugs

Lipids such as triglycerides and cholesterylesters are insoluble in water and are transported in plasma in the core of particles (**lipoproteins**) which have a hydrophilic shell of phospholipids and free cholesterol. This surface layer is stabilized by one or more **apolipoproteins** which also act as ligands for cell surface **receptors**. About two-thirds of plasma lipoproteins are synthesized in the liver (shaded). Triglycerides (TG) are secreted into the blood as *very low density lipoproteins* (*VLDL*) (⟹). In muscle and adipose tissue, the capillaries (right) possess an enzyme, *lipoprotein lipase* (), which hydrolyses the triglycerides to fatty acids; these then enter the muscle cells (for energy) and adipocytes (for storage). The residual particles containing a core rich in cholesterylester (CE) are called *low density lipoprotein* (*LDL*) particles. The liver and other cells possess *LDL receptors* () which remove LDL from the plasma by endocytosis (top figure). *The hepatic receptor mediated removal of LDL is the main mechanism for controlling plasma LDL levels.*

Fatty acids and cholesterol from ingested dietary fat are re-esterified in mucosal cells of the intestine and form the core of *chylomicrons* which enter the plasma via the thoracic duct. Fatty acids are hydrolysed

from the chylomicrons by lipoprotein lipase and the residual triglyceride-depleted *remnants* and are removed by the liver.

There is a strong positive correlation between the plasma concentration of LDL cholesterol and the development of **atherosclerosis** in medium and large arteries. Therapy that lowers LDL and raises high density lipoprotein (HDL) has been shown to reduce the progression of coronary atherosclerosis. **Lipid-lowering drugs** are indicated most strongly in patients with coronary artery disease, or those with high risk of coronary artery disease because of multiple **risk factors**, and in patients with familial hypercholesterolaemia. **Anion exchange resins** (top left, Ⓐ) bind bile acids () and since they are not absorbed, cholesterol excretion is increased. The **statins**, 3-hydroxy-3-methylglutaryl coenzyme A (**HMG CoA**) **reductase inhibitors** (top right), decrease hepatic cholesterol synthesis. The fall in hepatocyte cholesterol caused by resins and statins induces a compensatory increase in hepatic LDL receptors (top figure) and consequently a fall in plasma cholesterol. **Nicotinic acid** (centre right) reduces the release of VLDL by the liver whilst the **fibrates** (bottom right), which mainly lower triglyceride levels, probably act mainly by stimulating lipoprotein lipase.

Lipoproteins are classified according to their density on equilibrium ultracentrifugation. The larger particles (chylomicrons, remnants and VLDL) are the least dense and are not atherogenic because their greater size (30–500 nm diameter) prevents them passing into blood vessel walls. LDL particles (diameter 18–25 nm) can easily penetrate damaged arteries and are mainly responsible for the development of atherosclerosis. HDL particles are the smallest (diameter 5–12 nm) and epidemiological studies have revealed that high levels of HDL are associated with a lower incidence of atheroma. HDL accepts excess (unesterified) cholesterol from cells and also from lipoproteins which have lost their triglycerides and therefore have an excess of surface components, including cholesterol. The cholesterol is made less polar by re-esterification, causing it to move into the hydrophobic core and leaving the surface available to accept more cholesterol. The cholesterylesters are then returned to the liver. The removal of cholesterol from artery walls by HDL is thought to be the basis of its anti-atherogenic action.

Hyperlipidaemias. Primary lipoprotein disorders may involve cholesterol, triglycerides, or both. Secondary hyperlipidaemias are the result of another illness, e.g. diabetes mellitus, hypothyroidism. Hypercholesterolaemia is the most common disorder. About 5% of cases are familial but in most cases the cause is unknown. The main therapy for hyperlipidaemias, except for severe and hereditary types, is dietary modification (i.e. low fat and diet restriction to obtain ideal body weight).

Atherosclerosis. It is not fully understood how atheromatous plaques develop in arteries but turbulent flow is thought to initiate the process by causing focal damage to the intima. The plaques which protrude into the lumen are rich in cholesterol and have a lipid core covered by a fibrous cap. If the cap ruptures, the subintima acts as a focus for thrombosis, and occlusion of the artery may cause unstable angina, myocardial infarction or stroke. Epidemiological studies have shown a strong positive correlation between plasma cholesterol concentration (LDL) and coronary atherosclerosis, the incidence and severity of which is greatly increased by other risk factors including *cigarette smoking, hypertension, diabetes, family or personal history of premature heart disease, left ventricular hypertrophy.*

LIPID-LOWERING DRUGS

HMG CoA reductase inhibitors (**statins**) are the most recent lipid-lowering drugs. They are very effective in lowering total and LDL cholesterol and have been shown to reduce coronary events and total mortality. They have few side effects and are now usually the drugs of first choice. HMG CoA reductase inhibitors block the synthesis of cholesterol in the liver (which takes up most of the drug). This stimulates the expression of more enzyme, tending to restore cholesterol synthesis to normal even in the presence of the drug. However, this compensatory effect is incomplete and the reduction of cholesterol in the hepatocytes leads to an increased expression of LDL receptors, which increases the clearance of cholesterol from the plasma. Strong evidence that the statins lower plasma cholesterol, mainly by increasing the number of LDL receptors, is the failure of the drugs to work in patients with homozygous familial hypercholesterolaemia (who have no LDL receptors).

Adverse effects are rare, the main one being myopathy. *The incidence of myopathy is increased in patients given combined therapy with nicotinic acid or fibrates.* Statins should not be given during pregnancy because cholesterol is essential for normal foetal development.

Anion exchange resins. Cholestyramine and **colestipol** are powders taken with liquid. They increase the excretion of bile acids, causing more cholesterol to be converted to bile acids. The fall in hepatocyte cholesterol concentration causes compensatory increases in HMG CoA reductase activity and the number of LDL receptors. Since anion exchange resins do not work in patients with homozygous familial hypercholesterolaemia it seems that increased expression of hepatic LDL receptors is the main mechanism by which resins lower plasma cholesterol.

Adverse effects are confined to the gut, because the resins are not absorbed, and include bloating, abdominal discomfort, diarrhoea and constipation.

Nicotinic acid reduces the release of VLDL and therefore lowers plasma triglycerides (by 30–50%). It also lowers cholesterol (by 10–20%) and increases HDL. Nicotinic acid was the first lipid-lowering drug to reduce overall mortality in patients with coronary artery disease but its use is limited by unwanted effects that include prostaglandin-mediated flushing, dizziness and palpitations. Nicotinic acid is now mainly used in combination with an anion exchange resin in patients with familial hypercholesterolaemia.

Fibrates (e.g. **gemfibrozil**, **bezafibrate**) produce a modest decrease in LDL (about 10%) and increase in HDL (about 10%). In contrast, they cause a marked fall in plasma triglycerides (about 30%), apparently by stimulating lipoprotein lipase activity. Fibrates are first-line drugs in patients with very high plasma triglyceride levels who are at risk of pancreatitis.

Adverse effects. All the fibrates can cause a myositis-like syndrome. The incidence of myositis is increased by concurrent use of HMG CoA inhibitors and such combinations should be avoided.

Drug combinations. Severe hyperlipidaemia may require a combination of lipid-lowering drugs, e.g. an ion exchange resin with an HMG CoA reductase inhibitor.

21 Agents used in anaemias

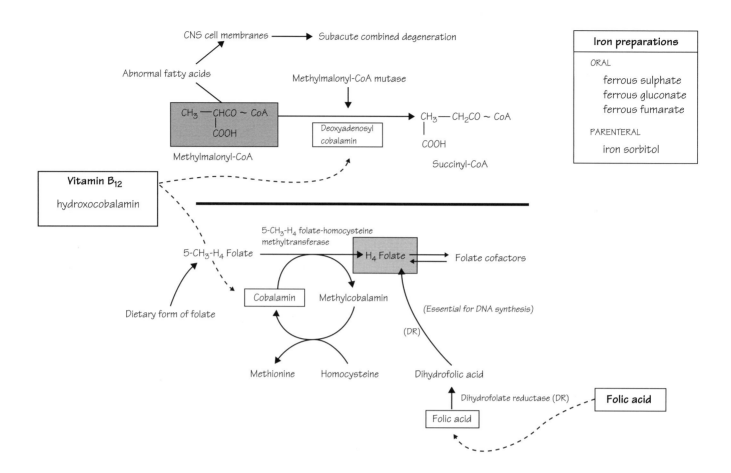

Normal erythropoiesis requires iron, vitamin B$_{12}$ and folic acid. A deficiency of any of these causes anaemia. Erythropoietic activity is regulated by **erythropoietin**, a hormone released mainly by the kidneys. In chronic renal failure, anaemia often occurs due to a fall in erythropoietin production.

Iron is necessary for haemoglobin production, and iron deficiency results in small red blood cells with insufficient haemoglobin (microcytic hypochromic anaemia). The administration of iron preparations (top right) is needed in iron deficiency, which may be due to chronic blood loss, pregnancy (the fetus takes iron from the mother), various abnormalities of the gut (iron absorption may be reduced) or premature birth (such babies are born with very low iron stores).

The main problem with oral iron preparations is that they frequently cause *gastrointestinal upsets*. Oral therapy is continued until haemoglobin is normal and the body stores of iron are built up by several months of lower iron doses. Children are very sensitive to iron toxicity and can be killed by as little as 1 g of ferrous sulphate. Overdosage of iron is treated with oral and parenteral **desferrioxamine**, a potent iron chelating agent.

Vitamin B$_{12}$ and **folic acid** are essential for several reactions necessary for normal DNA synthesis. A deficiency of either vitamin causes impaired production and abnormal maturation of erythroid precursor cells (megaloblastic anaemia). In addition to anaemia, vitamin B$_{12}$ deficiency causes *central nervous system degeneration* (subacute combined degeneration), which may result in psychiatric or physical symptoms. The anaemia is due to a block of H$_4$ folate synthesis (lower figure, �▮) and the nervous degeneration is due to an accumulation of methylmalonyl-CoA (upper figure, ▭).

Vitamin B$_{12}$ deficiency occurs when there is malabsorption due to lack of intrinsic factor (pernicious anaemia), following gastrectomy (no intrinsic factor), or in various small bowel diseases, where absorption is impaired. Since the disease is nearly always due to malabsorption, oral vitamin administration is of little value, and replacement therapy, usually for life, involves injections of vitamin B$_{12}$ (left). Hydroxocobalamin is the form of choice for therapy because it is retained in the body longer than cyanocobalamin (cyanocobalamin is bound less to plasma proteins and is more rapidly excreted in urine).

Folic acid deficiency leading to a megaloblastic anaemia, which requires oral folic acid (bottom right), may occur in pregnancy (folate requirement is increased) and in malabsorption syndromes (e.g. steatorrhoea and sprue).

IRON

The nucleus of haem is formed by iron, which, in combination with the appropriate globin chains, forms the protein haemoglobin. Over 90% of the non-storage iron in the body is in haemoglobin (about 2.3 g). Some iron (about 1 g) is stored as ferritin and haemosiderin in macrophages in the spleen, liver and bone marrow.

Absorption. Iron is normally absorbed in the duodenum and proximal jejunum. Normally 5–10% of dietary iron is absorbed (about 0.5–1 mg day^{-1}) but this can be increased if iron stores are low. Iron must be in the ferrous form for absorption, which occurs by active transport. In the plasma, iron is transported bound to transferrin, a β-globulin. There is no mechanism for excretion of iron and regulation of iron balance is achieved by appropriate changes in iron absorption.

IRON PREPARATIONS

For oral therapy iron preparations contain ferrous salts because these are absorbed most efficiently. In iron-deficient patients, about 50–100 mg of iron can be incorporated into haemoglobin daily. Since about 25% of oral ferrous salts can be absorbed, 200–400 mg iron should be given daily for the fastest possible correction of deficiency. If this causes intolerable gastrointestinal irritation (nausea, epigastric pain, diarrhoea, constipation), lower doses can be given; these will completely correct the iron deficiency, but more slowly.

Parenteral iron should only be used if oral therapy has failed. It does not hasten the haemoglobin response.

Iron sorbitol is a complex of iron, sorbitol and citric acid. It is not suitable for intravenous injection and is given by deep intramuscular injections to minimize staining of the skin. Parenteral iron may cause anaphylactoid reactions.

Iron toxicity. Acute toxicity occurs most commonly in young children who have ingested iron tablets. These cause necrotizing gastroenteritis with abdominal pain, vomiting, bloody diarrhoea and, later, shock. This may be followed, even after apparent improvement, by acidosis, coma and death.

VITAMIN B$_{12}$

In megaloblastic anaemias, the underlying defect is impaired DNA synthesis. Cell division is decreased but RNA and protein synthesis continue. This results in large (macrocytic) fragile red cells. The cobalt atom at the centre of the vitamin B$_{12}$ molecule covalently binds different ligands, forming various cobalamins. *Methylcobalamin* and *deoxyadenosylcobalamin* are the active forms of the vitamin and other cobalamins must be converted to these active forms.

Vitamin B$_{12}$ (extrinsic factor) is absorbed only when complexed with *intrinsic factor*, a glycoprotein secreted by the *parietal cells* of the gastric mucosa. Absorption occurs in the distal ileum by a highly spe-cific transport process and the vitamin is then transported bound to transcobalamin II (a plasma glycoprotein). *Pernicious anaemia* results from a *deficiency* in intrinsic factor caused by autoantibodies, either to the factor itself or to the gastric parietal cells (atrophic gastritis).

Methylmalonyl-CoA mutase. This enzyme requires deoxyadenosyl-cobalamin for the conversion of methylmalonyl-CoA to succinyl-CoA. In the absence of vitamin B$_{12}$, this reaction cannot take place and there is accumulation of *methylmalonyl-CoA*. This results in the synthesis of abnormal fatty acids, which become incorporated in neuronal membranes and cause the neurological defects seen in vitamin B$_{12}$ deficiency.

5-CH$_3$-H$_4$ folate-homocysteine methyltransferase converts 5-CH$_3$-H$_4$ folate and homocysteine to H$_4$ folate and methionine. In this reaction, cobalamin is converted to methylcobalamin. When vitamin B$_{12}$ deficiency prevents this reaction, the conversion of the major dietary and storage folate (5-CH$_3$-H$_4$ folate) to the precursor of folate cofactors (H$_4$ folate) cannot occur and a deficiency in the folate cofactors necessary for DNA synthesis develops. This reaction links folic acid and vitamin B$_{12}$ metabolism and explains why high doses of folic acid can improve the anaemia, but not the nervous degeneration, caused by vitamin B$_{12}$ deficiency.

FOLIC ACID

The body stores of folates are relatively low (5–20 mg) and as daily requirements are high, folic acid deficiency and megaloblastic anaemia can quickly develop (1–6 months) if the intake of folic acid stops. Folic acid itself is completely absorbed in the proximal jejunum, but dietary folates are mainly polyglutamate forms of 5-CH$_3$-H$_4$ folate. All but one of the glutamyl residues are hydrolysed off before the absorption of monoglutamate 5-CH$_3$-H$_4$ folate. In contrast to vitamin B$_{12}$ deficiency, folic acid deficiency is often caused by inadequate dietary intake of folate. Some drugs (e.g. *phenytoin, oral contraceptives, isoniazid*) can cause folic acid deficiency by reducing its absorption.

Folic acid and vitamin B$_{12}$ have no known toxic effects. However, it is important not to give folic acid alone in vitamin B$_{12}$ deficiency states, because although the anaemia may improve, the neurological degeneration progresses and may become irreversible.

ERYTHROPOIETIN

Hypoxia, or loss of blood, results in increased haemoglobin synthesis and release of erythrocytes. These changes are mediated by an increase in circulating erythropoietin (a glycoprotein containing 166 amino acid residues). Erythropoietin binds to receptors on erythroid cell precursors in the bone marrow and increases the transcription of enzymes involved in haem synthesis. Recombinant erythropoietin (**epoetin**) (given by intravenous or subcutaneous injection) is used to correct anaemia in chronic renal failure disease, which is caused largely by a deficiency of the hormone.

22 Central transmitter substances

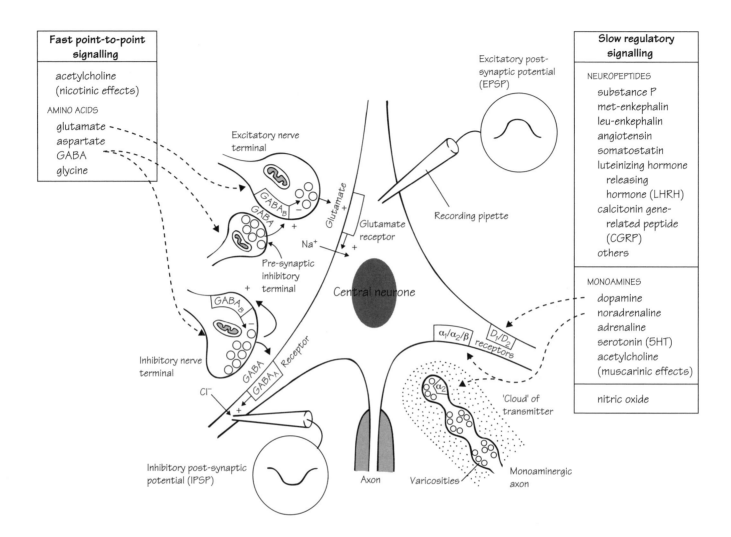

Fast point-to-point signalling
- acetylcholine (nicotinic effects)
- AMINO ACIDS
  - glutamate
  - aspartate
  - GABA
  - glycine

Slow regulatory signalling
- NEUROPEPTIDES
  - substance P
  - met-enkephalin
  - leu-enkephalin
  - angiotensin
  - somatostatin
  - luteinizing hormone releasing hormone (LHRH)
  - calcitonin gene-related peptide (CGRP)
  - others
- MONOAMINES
  - dopamine
  - noradrenaline
  - adrenaline
  - serotonin (5HT)
  - acetylcholine (muscarinic effects)
- nitric oxide

Drugs acting on the central nervous system are used more than any other type of agent. In addition to their therapeutic uses, drugs such as **caffeine**, **alcohol** and **nicotine** are used socially to provide a sense of well-being. Central drugs often produce dependence with continued use (Chapter 31) and many are subject to strict legal controls.

The mechanisms by which central drugs produce their therapeutic effects are usually unknown, reflecting our lack of understanding of neurological and psychiatric disease. Knowledge of central transmitter substances is important because virtually all drugs acting on the brain produce their effects by modifying synaptic transmission.

The transmitters used in fast, point-to-point neural circuits are **amino acids** (left), except for a few cholinergic synapses with nicotinic receptors. **Glutamate** is the main central excitatory transmitter. It depolarizes neurones by triggering an increase in membrane Na^+ conductance. **γ-Aminobutyric acid (GABA)** is the main inhibitory transmitter, perhaps being released at one-third of all central synapses. It hyperpolarizes neurones by increasing their membrane Cl^- conductance and stabilizes the resting membrane potential near the Cl^- equi-

librium potential. *Glycine* is also an inhibitory transmitter, mainly in the spinal cord.

In addition to fast point-to-point signalling, the brain possesses more diffuse regulatory systems, which use **monoamines** as their transmitters (bottom right). The cell bodies of these branched axons project to many areas of the brain. Transmitter release occurs diffusely from many points along varicose terminal networks of monoaminergic neurones, affecting very large numbers of target cells. The functions of the central monoaminergic pathways are obscure, but they are involved in disorders such as *Parkinsonism, depression, migraine* and *schizophrenia*.

Many **peptides** (top right) have been found in central neurones and nerve terminals. The evidence for their role as transmitter substances is usually very incomplete. They probably form another group of diffusely acting regulatory transmitters, but as yet the physiological roles of most of them are unknown.

Most recently, it has been suggested that **nitric oxide** (NO) might act as a transmitter in the brain.

AMINO ACIDS

γ-Aminobutyric acid is present in all areas of the central nervous system, mainly in local inhibitory interneurones. It rapidly inhibits central neurones, the response being mediated by postsynaptic GABA$_A$ receptors, which are blocked by the convulsant drug bicuculline. Some GABA receptors (GABA$_B$) are not blocked by bicuculline, but are selectively activated by **baclofen** (*p*-chlorophenyl-GABA). Many GABA$_B$ receptors are located on presynaptic nerve terminals and their activation results in a reduction in transmitter release (e.g. of glutamate and GABA itself). Baclofen reduces glutamate release in the spinal cord and produces an antispastic effect, which is useful in controlling the muscular spasms that occur in diseases such as multiple sclerosis.

Following release from presynaptic nerve terminals, amino acid transmitters are inactivated by reuptake systems.

Drugs which are thought to act by modifying GABAergic synaptic transmission include the **benzodiazepines, barbiturates** (Chapter 24) and the anticonvulsants **vigabatrin** and perhaps **valproate** (Chapter 25).

Glycine is an inhibitory transmitter in spinal interneurones. It is antagonized by strychnine and its release is prevented by tetanus toxin, both substances causing convulsions.

Glutamate excites virtually all central neurones by activating several types of excitatory amino acid receptor. These receptors are classified into (ligand-gated) kainate, AMPA* and NMDA* receptors, depending whether or not they are selectively activated by these glutamate analogues. A family of metabotropic (G-protein coupled) receptors also exists. NMDA receptor antagonists (e.g. 2-aminophosphonovalerate) have been shown to have anticonvulsant activity in many experimental animal models of epilepsy and they may prove to be beneficial in stroke, where at least some of the neuronal damage is thought to result from an excessive release of glutamate. Lamotrigine is an antiepileptic drug (Chapter 25) that is thought to act, at least partly, by reducing presynaptic glutamate release.

MONOAMINES

Acetylcholine is mainly excitatory in the brain. It is the transmitter released from motoneurone nerve endings at the neuromuscular junction and at collateral axon synapses with Renshaw cells in the spinal cord. This provides the best example of a central nicotinic synapse. The excitatory effects of acetylcholine on central neurones are usually mediated via muscarinic receptors and may involve suppression of a voltage-sensitive K$^+$ conductance (M current). This inhibition increases the excitability of the cell and facilitates its response to tonic excitatory influences.

Cholinergic neurones are particularly abundant in the basal ganglia and others seem to be involved in cortical arousal responses and in memory. **Atropine-like** drugs can impair memory and the amnesic

action of hyoscine is made use of in anaesthetic premedication (Chapter 23). They are also used for their central actions in *motion sickness* and *Parkinsonism* (Chapter 26). Loss of cholinergic neurones and memory are prominant features of *Alzheimer's disease*, a common form of senile dementia for which there is no effective treatment at present. **Tacrine** is an anticholinesterase of modest benefit to some (*c.* 15%) patients with Alzheimer's disease but is hepatotoxic.

Catecholamines generally have inhibitory effects when applied locally to central neurones.

Dopamine pathways project from the *substantia nigra* in the midbrain to the basal ganglia and from the *midbrain* to the limbic cortex and other limbic structures. A third (tuberoinfundibular) pathway is involved in regulating prolactin release. The nigrostriatal pathway is concerned with modulating the control of voluntary movement and its degeneration results in *Parkinsonism*. The mesolimbic pathway is 'overactive' in *schizophrenia*, but it is not known why. Dopamine *agonists* are used in the treatment of Parkinsonism (Chapter 26) and *antagonists* (neuroleptics) are used in schizophrenia (Chapter 27). The chemoreceptor trigger zone (CTZ) has dopamine receptors, and dopamine antagonists have *anti-emetic* effects (Chapter 30).

Noradrenaline-containing cell bodies occur in several groups in the brainstem. The largest of these nuclei is the *locus coeruleus* in the pons, which projects to the entire dorsal forebrain, especially the cerebral cortex and hippocampus. The hypothalamus also possesses a high density of noradrenergic fibres. Noradrenaline and dopamine in limbic forebrain structures (especially the nucleus accumbens) may be involved in an ascending 'reward' system which has been implicated in *drug dependence* (Chapter 31). Impairment of noradrenergic function may be associated with *depression* (Chapter 28).

Serotonin (5-hydroxytryptamine, 5HT) occurs in cell bodies in the *raphe nucleus* of the brainstem which projects to many forebrain areas and to the ventral and dorsal horns of the spinal cord. The latter, descending projection may modulate pain inputs (Chapter 29). 5HT may, like noradrenaline, be involved in *depression*. 5HT$_3$ receptors occur in the CTZ and antagonists have antiemetic effects. 5HT$_{1D}$ receptors occur in cranial blood vessels and the agonist **sumatriptan** relieves migraine by constricting the vessels that are abnormally dilated during the attack.

Neuropeptides form the most numerous group of possible central transmitters, but little is known yet of their functions. Substance P and the enkephalins are thought to be involved in pain pathways (Chapter 29).

NO. Nitric oxide synthase (NOS) is present in about 1–2% of neurones in many areas of the brain, e.g. cerebral cortex, hippocampus, striatum. NOS has been found colocalized with other transmitters, e.g. GABA, glutamate, somatostatin, neuropeptide Y, and NO affects the release of other transmitters. The physiological roles of NO in the brain are unknown but there is evidence that it may be involved in synaptic plasticity, e.g. long-term potentiation.

---

*AMPA, α-amino-3-hydroxy-5-methyl-4-isoxazolepropionic acid; NMDA, *N*-methyl-D-aspartate.

23 General anaesthetics

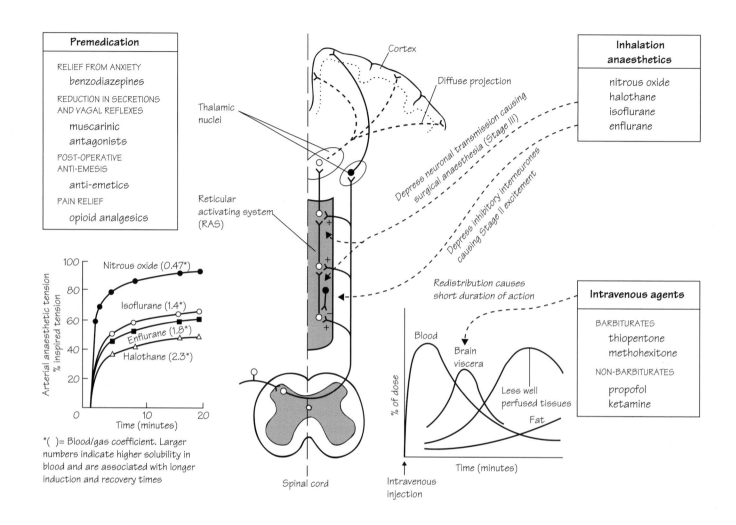

Premedication

RELIEF FROM ANXIETY
benzodiazepines

REDUCTION IN SECRETIONS AND VAGAL REFLEXES
muscarinic antagonists

POST-OPERATIVE ANTI-EMESIS
anti-emetics

PAIN RELIEF
opioid analgesics

Inhalation anaesthetics

nitrous oxide
halothane
isoflurane
enflurane

Intravenous agents

BARBITURATES
thiopentone
methohexitone

NON-BARBITURATES
propofol
ketamine

Cortex
Diffuse projection
Thalamic nuclei
Reticular activating system (RAS)
Spinal cord

Depress neuronal transmission causing surgical anaesthesia (Stage III)
Depress inhibitory interneurones causing Stage II excitement
Redistribution causes short duration of action

Nitrous oxide (0.47*)
Isoflurane (1.4*)
Enflurane (1.8*)
Halothane (2.3*)

Arterial anaesthetic tension % inspired tension
Time (minutes)

*( ) = Blood/gas coefficient. Larger numbers indicate higher solubility in blood and are associated with longer induction and recovery times

Blood
Brain viscera
Less well perfused tissues
Fat
% of dose
Time (minutes)
Intravenous injection

General anaesthesia is the absence of sensation associated with a reversible loss of consciousness. Numerous agents ranging from inert gases to steroids produce anaesthesa in animals, but only a few are used clinically (right). Historical anaesthetics include ether, chloroform, cyclopropane, ethylchloride and trichlorethylene.

Anaesthetics depress all excitable tissues including central neurones, cardiac muscle and smooth and striatal muscle. However, these tissues have different sensitivities to anaesthetics and the areas of the brain responsible for consciousness (middle, ▭) are among the most sensitive. Thus, it is possible to administer anaesthetic agents at concentrations that produce unconsciousness without unduly depressing the cardiovascular and respiratory centres or the myocardium. However, for most anaesthetics, *the margin of safety is small.*

General anaesthesia usually involves the administration of different drugs for:
- **premedication** (top left),
- **induction** of anaesthesia (bottom right) and
- **maintenance** of anaesthesia (top right). Premedication has two main aims:

1 the prevention of the parasympathomimetic effects of anaesthesia (bradycardia, bronchial secretion); and

2 the reduction of anxiety or pain.

Premedication is often omitted for minor operations. If necessary, the appropriate drugs (e.g. hyoscine) are given intravenously at induction.

Induction is most commonly achieved by the intravenous injection of **thiopentone** or **propofol**. Unconsciousness occurs within seconds and is maintained by the administration of an inhalation anaesthetic. **Halothane** is a widely used volatile anaesthetic in the UK, but it is associated with a very low incidence of postoperative hepatitis. **Enflurane** and **isoflurane** are newer agents that are being used increasingly because they are not hepatotoxic. **Nitrous oxide** at concentrations up to 70% in oxygen is the most widely used anaesthetic agent. It is used with oxygen as a carrier gas, for the volatile agents, or together with opioid analgesics (e.g. *fentanyl*). Nitrous oxide causes sedation and analgesia but it is not sufficient alone to maintain anaesthesia.

During the induction of anaesthesia, distinct 'stages' occur with some agents, especially ether. First, analgesia is produced (stage I), followed by excitement (stage II) caused by inhibition of inhibitory reticular neurones (○—<). Then surgical anaesthesia (stage III) develops, the depth of which depends on the amount of drug administered. These stages are not obvious with currently used anaesthetics.

Reticular activating system (RAS). This is a complex polysynaptic pathway in the brainstem reticular formation that projects diffusely to the cortex. Activity in the RAS is concerned with maintaining consciousness and, because it is especially sensitive to the depressant action of anaesthetics, it is thought to be their primary site of action.

Mechanism of action of anaesthetics. It is not known how anaesthetics produce their effects. Anaesthetic potency correlates well with lipid solubility and anaesthetics may dissolve in the lipid bilayer of the cell membrane, expanding the membrane and increasing its fluidity. The resulting disorder in the membrane may alter ionic fluxes (decrease sodium influx or increase potassium efflux) and produce anaesthesia. A finding consistent with this idea is that high pressure reverses anaesthesia, presumably by 'reordering' the cell membrane. Another possibility is that anaesthetics might bind to a hydrophobic area of a protein and inhibit its normal function.

PREMEDICATION

Relief from anxiety (Chapter 24). Oral **benzodiazepines** such as diazepam or lorazepam are most effective.

Reduction in secretions and vagal reflexes. Muscarinic antagonists, usually **atropine** or **hyoscine**, are used to prevent salivation and bronchial secretions and, more importantly, to protect the heart from arrhythmias, particularly bradycardia caused by halothane, suxamethonium and neostigmine. Hyoscine is also anti-emetic and produces some amnesia.

Analgesics. Opioid analgesics, e.g. morphine (Chapter 29), may be given before an operation but this is not a logical choice of drug unless the patient is in pain. **Fentanyl** and related drugs (e.g **alfentanyl**) are used intravenously to supplement nitrous oxide anaesthesia. These opioids are highly lipid soluble and have a rapid onset of action. They have a short duration of action because of redistribution.

Postoperative anti-emesis. Nausea and vomiting are very common after anaesthesia. Often, opioid drugs given during and after the operation are responsible. Sometimes anti-emetic drugs (e.g.**metoclopramide**, **ondansetron**) are given with the premedication, but they are more effective if administered intravenously during anaesthesia.

INTRAVENOUS AGENTS

These may be used alone for short surgical procedures, but are used mainly for the induction of anaesthesia.

Barbiturates. Thiopentone injected intravenously induces anaesthesia in less than 30 seconds because the very lipid-soluble drug quickly dissolves in the rapidly perfused brain. Recovery from thiopentone is rapid because of redistribution into less-perfused tissues (bottom right figure). Thiopentone is subsequently metabolized by the liver at a rate of 12–16% per hour. Doses of thiopentone only slightly above the 'sleep dose' depress the myocardium and the respiratory centre. Very occasionally anaphylaxis may occur.

Non-barbiturates. Many agents with potential advantages over the barbiturates (e.g. less myocardial depression, more rapid elimination) have been introduced, but few have found much favour for long. **Propofol** (2,6-diisopropylphenol) is associated with rapid recovery without nausea or hangover and for this reason is widely used. It may, however, occasionally cause convulsions and, very rarely, anaphylaxis. **Ketamine** may be given by intramuscular or intravenous injection. It is analgesic in subanaesthetic doses but often causes hallucinations. Its main use is in paediatric anaesthesia.

INHALATION AGENTS

Uptake and distribution (bottom left figure). The speed at which induction of anaesthesia occurs depends mainly on its *solubility in blood* and the *inspired concentration* of gas. When agents of low solubility (nitrous oxide) diffuse from the lungs into arterial blood, relatively small amounts are required to saturate the blood, and so the arterial tension (and hence brain tension) rises quickly. More soluble agents (halothane) require the solution of much more anaesthetic before the arterial anaesthetic tension approaches that of the inspired gas and so induction is slower. Recovery from anaesthesia is also slower with increasing anaesthetic solubility.

Nitrous oxide is not potent enough to use as a sole anaesthetic agent, but it is commonly used as a non-flammable carrier gas for volatile agents, allowing their concentration to be significantly reduced. It is a good analgesic and a 50% mixture in oxygen (Entonox) is used when analgesia is required (e.g. in childbirth, road traffic accidents). Nitrous oxide has little effect on the cardiovascular or respiratory systems.

Halothane ($CF_3CHBrCl$) is a potent agent and, as the vapour is non-irritant, induction is smooth and pleasant. It causes a concentration-dependent hypotension, largely by myocardial depression. Halothane often causes arrhythmias and because the myocardium is sensitized to catecholamines, infiltration of adrenaline may cause cardiac arrest. Like most volatile anaesthetics, halothane depresses the respiratory centre, with a resulting decrease in the minute volume and an increase in arterial P_{CO_2}. The most important toxic effect of halothane is massive hepatic necrosis, which occurs in about 1 in 35 000 cases, although lesser degrees of liver damage probably occur much more often. More than 20% of the administered halothane is biotransformed by the liver to metabolites, some of which may either directly damage the liver or bind to cellular macromolecules and generate antigens that are recognized as foreign by the body. Severe hepatotoxicity is more likely after repeated exposure to halothane, which should be avoided.

Enflurane ($F_2HC–O–CF_2–CHFCl$) is similar in action to halothane. It undergoes much less metabolism (2%) than halothane and is unlikely to cause hepatitis. The disadvantage of enflurane is that it may cause seizure activity in the electroencephalogram (EEG) and, occasionally, muscle twitching.

Isoflurane ($F_3CCHCl–O–CF_2H$) has similar actions to halothane but is less cardiodepressant and does not sensitize the heart to adrenaline. It causes dose-related hypotension by decreasing systemic vascular resistance. Only 0.2% of the absorbed dose is metabolized and so isoflurane is very unlikely to cause hepatitis.

24 Anxiolytics and hypnotics

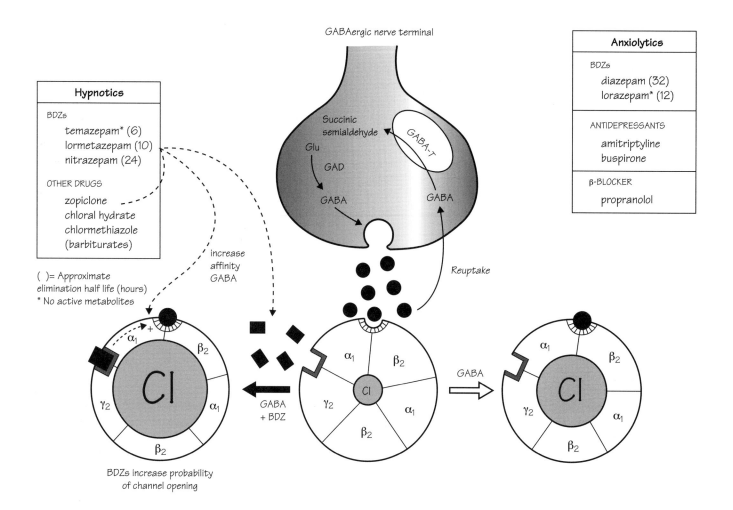

Hypnotics

BDZs
  temazepam* (6)
  lormetazepam (10)
  nitrazepam (24)

OTHER DRUGS
  zopiclone
  chloral hydrate
  chlormethiazole
  (barbiturates)

( ) = Approximate elimination half life (hours)
* No active metabolites

GABAergic nerve terminal

Succinic semialdehyde
Glu
GAD
GABA
GABA-T
GABA
Reuptake

increase affinity GABA

GABA + BDZ

GABA

BDZs increase probability of channel opening

Anxiolytics

BDZs
  diazepam (32)
  lorazepam* (12)

ANTIDEPRESSANTS
  amitriptyline
  buspirone

β-BLOCKER
  propranolol

Drug treatment of *sleep disorders* (hypnotics) and *acute anxiety states* (anxiolytics) is dominated by the **benzodiazepines** (BDZs). In general, these drugs will induce sleep when given in high doses at night and will provide sedation and reduce anxiety when given in low, divided doses during the day.

BDZs have *anxiolytic, hypnotic, muscle relaxant* and *anticonvulsant* (Chapter 25) actions which are thought to be caused mainly by the enhancement of *GABA-mediated inhibition* in the central nervous system. GABA (●) released from nerve terminals (top middle, shaded) binds to **GABA$_A$ receptors** ( ), the activation of which increases the Cl$^-$ conductance of the neurone (bottom right). The GABA$_A$/Cl$^-$ channel complex also has a BDZ modulatory receptor site ( ). Occupation of the BDZ sites by BDZ receptor agonists (■) causes a conformational change in the GABA receptor. This increases the affinity of GABA binding and enhances the actions of GABA on the Cl$^-$ conductance of the neuronal membrane (bottom left). The **barbiturates** act at another binding site and similarly enhance the action of GABA (not illustrated). In the absence of GABA, BDZs and low doses of barbiturates do not affect Cl$^-$ conductance.

The popularity of BDZs arose from their apparently low toxicity, but it is now realized that chronic BDZ treatment may cause cognitive impairment, tolerance and **dependence**. For these reasons BDZs should only be used for 2–4 weeks to treat severe anxiety and insomnia.

Many **antidepressants** (e.g. **amitriptyline**) are also anxiolytic and do not cause dependence. **Buspirone** is a non-sedative anxiolytic that acts at 5HT synapses.

Different benzodiazepines are marketed as hypnotics (top left) and anxiolytics (top right). It is mainly the duration of action that determines the choice of drug. Many BDZs are metabolized in the liver to **active metabolites**, which may have longer elimination half-lives ($t_{1/2}$) than the parent drug. For example, **diazepam** ($t_{1/2}$; ≈ 20–80 hours) has an active *N*-desmethyl metabolite that has an elimination half-life of up to 200 hours.

BDZs used as hypnotics (top left) can be divided into short acting and longer acting. A rapidly eliminated drug (e.g. **temazepam**) is usually preferred to avoid daytime sedation. A longer-acting drug (e.g. **nitrazepam**) might be preferred where early morning waking is a problem and where a daytime anxiolytic effect is needed. **Zopiclone** acts at benzodiazepine receptors but is a cyclopyrrolone. This more recent drug has a short duration of action.

GABA receptors (Chapter 22) of the GABA$_A$ type are involved in the actions of hypnotics/anxiolytics. The GABA$_A$ receptor belongs to the superfamily of ligand-gated ion channels (other examples are the nicotinic, glycine and 5HT$_3$ receptors). The GABA$_A$ receptor consists of several subunits (α, β, γ and δ) and variants of each of these subunits have been cloned (six α-, four β-, four γ- and two δ- subunits). The subunit compositions of natural GABA$_A$ receptors in the brain are unknown. If the GABA$_A$ receptor is pentameric (like the nicotinic receptor), then a major type is probably $2\alpha_1\,2\beta_2,\,\gamma_2$ because mRNAs encoding these subunits are often colocalized in the brain. Electrophysiological experiments on toad oocytes possessing various combinations of GABA$_A$ subunits (produced by injecting their mRNA into the oocyte) have revealed that receptors constructed from α- and β-subunits respond to GABA (i.e. the Cl$^-$ conductance increases), but for a receptor to respond fully to a BDZ, a γ$_2$-subunit is required. Recent photoaffinity experiments suggest that the BDZ and GABA binding sites are partially colocated on an α-subunit (bottom figure).

Recently, compounds have been discovered that are *antagonists* or *partial agonists* at the BDZ receptors. Others actually increase anxiety and are called *inverse agonists*. It remains to be seen whether the development of partial agonists will lead to a non-sedative anxiolytic.

Flumazenil is a competitive BDZ antagonist that has a short duration of action and is given intravenously. It can be used to reverse the sedative effects of BDZs in anaesthetic, intensive care, diagnostic procedures, and in overdoses.

Barbiturate receptor. Barbiturates increase GABA-mediated inhibition by prolonging the duration of individual Cl$^-$ channel openings triggered by a given GABA stimulus (BDZs increase the frequency of Cl$^-$ channel opening). Barbiturates are far more depressant than BDZs, because at higher doses they increase the Cl$^-$ conductance directly and decrease the sensitivity of the neuronal postsynaptic membrane to excitatory transmitters.

Barbiturates were extensively used but are now obsolete as hypnotics and anxiolytics because they readily lead to psychological and physical dependence, induce microsomal enzymes, and relatively small overdosage may be fatal. In contrast, huge overdoses of BDZs have been taken without serious long-term effects. Barbiturates (e.g. **thiopentone**, Chapter 23) remain important in anaesthesia and are still used as anticonvulsants (e.g. **phenobarbitone**, Chapter 25).

BDZs

These are active orally and although most are metabolized by oxidation in the liver, they do not induce hepatic enzyme systems. They are central depressants, but in contrast to other hypnotics and anxiolytics, their maximum effect when given orally does not normally cause fatal, or even severe, respiratory depression. However, respiratory depression may occur in patients with bronchopulmonary disease or with intravenous administration.

Adverse effects include drowsiness, impaired alertness, agitation and ataxia, especially in the elderly.

Dependence. A physical withdrawal syndrome may occur in patients given BDZs for even short periods. The symptoms, which may persist for weeks or months, include anxiety, insomnia, depression, nausea and perceptual changes.

Drug interactions. BDZs have additive or synergistic effects with other central depressants such as alcohol, barbiturates and antihistamines.

Intravenous BDZs (e.g. **diazepam, clonazepam**) are used in status epilepticus (Chapter 25) and very occasionally in panic attacks (however, oral **alprazolam** is probably more effective for this latter purpose and is safer). **Midazolam**, unlike other BDZs, forms water-soluble salts and is used as an intravenous sedative during endoscopic and dental procedures. When given intravenously BDZs have an impressive amnesic action and patients may remember nothing of unpleasant procedures.

ANTIDEPRESSANTS

Tricyclic antidepressants, such as **amitriptyline**, have anxiolytic effects. They are used in patients with depression and anxiety, and for patients who require long-term anxiolytic drugs where BDZs would result in dependence. Monoamine oxidase inhibitors may be especially useful in phobic anxiety disorders (Chapter 28).

DRUGS ACTING AT SEROTONERGIC (5HT) RECEPTORS

5HT cell bodies are located in the raphé nuclei of the mid brain and project to many areas of the brain including those thought to be important in anxiety (hippocampus, amygdala, frontal cortex). In rats, lesions of the raphé nuclei produce anxiolytic effects, whilst stimulation of 5HT receptors with agonists produce anxiogenic effects. A role for 5HT in anxiety was strengthened when it was found that BDZs micro-injected into the dorsal raphé nucleus reduce the rate of neuronal firing and produce an anxiolytic effect. These experiments suggested that 5HT antagonists might be useful anxiolytic drugs. Antagonists at 5HT$_3$ receptors (e.g. ondansetron) and 5HT$_2$ receptors (e.g. ritanserin) have little, if any, anxiolytic action. However, **buspirone**, a 5HT$_{1A}$ partial agonist, has anxiolytic actions in humans, perhaps by acting as an antagonist at postsynaptic 5HT$_{1A}$ sites in the hippocampus (where there is little receptor reserve). Buspirone is not sedative and does not cause dependence. Unfortunately, it is only anxiolytic after 2 weeks' administration and the indications for buspirone are unclear.

β-**Adrenoceptor blockers**, such as propranolol, can be very effective in alleviating the autonomic symptoms of anxiety such as tremor, palpitations, sweating and diarrhoea.

Chloral hydrate is converted in the body to trichloroethanol, which is an effective hypnotic. It is cheap but may cause gastric irritation. *Dichloralphenazone* is a derivative of chloral hydrate that is not a gastric irritant. These drugs are useful in the young and elderly. They can cause tolerance and dependence.

Chlormethiazole has no advantage over short-acting BDZs, except in the elderly, where it may cause less hangover. It is given by intravenous infusion in cases of acute alcohol withdrawal and in status epilepticus. Chlormethiazole causes dependence and should be used only for a limited period.

25 Antiepileptic drugs

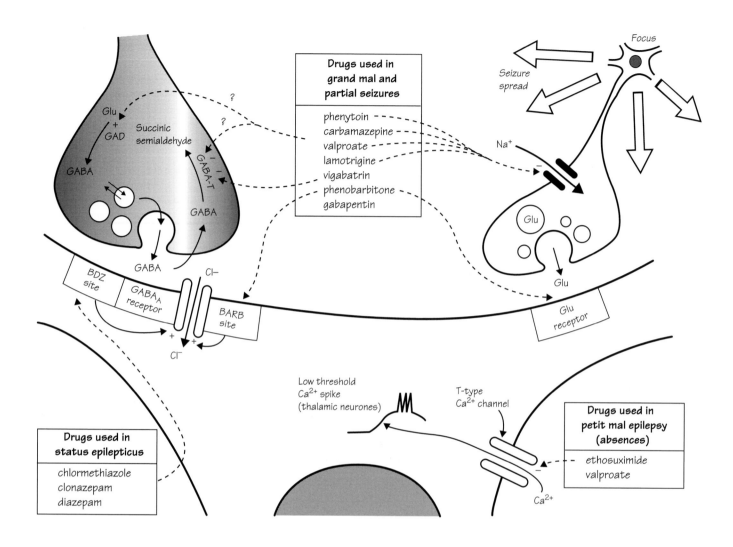

Epilepsy is a chronic disease in which seizures result from the abnormal discharge of cerebral neurones. The seizures are classified empirically.

Partial (focal) seizures begin at a specific locus (upper right figure) in the brain and may be limited to clonic jerking of an extremity. However, the discharge may spread (⟳) and become generalized (**secondarily generalized seizure**). **Generalized seizures** are those in which there is no evidence of localized onset, both cerebral hemispheres being involved from the onset. They include **tonic–clonic** attacks (*grand mal*—periods of tonic rigidity followed later by massive jerking of the body) and **absences** (*petit mal*—changes in consciousness usually lasting less than 10 seconds).

Tonic–clonic and partial seizures are treated mainly with oral **carbamazepine** (top middle), **phenytoin** or **valproate**. These drugs are of similar effectiveness and a single drug will control the fits in 70–80% of patients with tonic–clonic seizures, but only 30–40% of patients with partial seizures. In these poorly controlled patients the addition of **lamotrigine**, **vigabatrin** or **gabapentin** may reduce the incidence of seizures, but only about 7% of these refractory patients become totally seizure free. **Phenobarbitone**, primidone and clonazepam are alterna-

tive drugs, but are more sedative.

Absence seizures are treated with **ethosuximide** (bottom right) or valproate. Petit mal only occasionally continues into adult life, but about 50% of children will later develop grand mal fits.

Status epilepticus is a state in which fits follow each other without consciousness being regained. Urgent treatment with intravenous agents (bottom left) is necessary to stop the fits, which, if unchecked, result in exhaustion and cerebral damage. Clonazepam or diazepam may be effective, but a continuous infusion of chlormethiazole is the treatment of choice.

Antiepileptic drugs control seizures by mechanisms that are often unclear, but usually involve either the enhancement of GABA-mediated inhibition (benzodiazepines, vigabatrin, phenobarbitone, valproate) (left of figure) or a reduction of Na$^+$ fluxes (phenytoin, carbamazepine, valproate, lamotrigine) (right figure). Ethosuximide and valproate may inhibit a spike-generating Ca^{2+} current in thalamic neurones (bottom right).

CAUSES OF EPILEPSY

The aetiology is unknown in 60–70% of cases, but heredity is an important factor. Damage to the brain, for example tumours, asphyxia, infections or head injury, may subsequently cause epilepsy. Convulsions may be precipitated in epileptics by several groups of drugs, including *phenothiazines*, *tricyclic antidepressants* and many *antihistamines*.

MECHANISMS OF ACTION OF ANTICONVULSANTS

The most-studied agent is **phenytoin**, which at therapeutic concentrations has no effect on transmitter release or on neuronal responses to glutamate or GABA. Its anticonvulsant action is probably due to its ability to *prevent high-frequency repetitive activity*. Just how phenytoin does this is not clear, but in voltage clamp experiments it has been shown to increase the proportion of inactivated Na^+ channels for any given membrane potential. Phenytoin binds preferentially to inactivated (closed) Na^+ channels, stabilizing them in the inactivated state and preventing them from returning to the resting (closed) state that they must re-enter before they can again open (see Chapter 5). High frequency repetitive depolarization increases the proportion of Na^+ channels in the inactivated state and because these are susceptible to blockade by phenytoin, the Na^+ current is progressively reduced until it is eventually insufficient to evoke an action potential. Neuronal transmission at normal frequencies is relatively unaffected by phenytoin, because a much smaller proportion of the Na^+ channels are in the inactivated state. **Carbamazepine**, **lamotrigine** and **valproate** have similar actions on neuronal Na^+ channels. Valproate also seems to increase GABAergic central inhibition by mechanisms that may involve stimulation of glutamic acid decarboxylase activity and/or inhibition of GABA-T activity. **Vigabatrin** is an irreversible inhibitor of GABA-T, which increases brain GABA levels and central GABA release. The benzodiazepines (e.g. **clonazepam**) and **phenobarbitone** also increase central inhibition, but by enhancing the action of synaptically released GABA at the $GABA_A$ receptor–Cl^- channel complex (Chapter 24). Phenobarbitone may also reduce the effects of glutamate at excitatory synapses.

Absence seizures involve oscillatory neuronal activity between the thalamus and cerebral cortex. This oscillation involves (T-type) Ca^{2+} channels in the thalamic neurones, which produce low threshold spikes and allow the cells to fire in bursts. Recent evidence suggests that drugs that control absences (**ethosuxamide** and **valproate**) reduce this Ca^{2+} current, dampening the thalamocortical oscillations that are critical in the generation of absence seizures.

DRUGS USED IN PARTIAL AND GRAND MAL SEIZURES

Treatment with a single drug is preferred because this reduces adverse effects and drug interactions. Furthermore, most patients obtain no extra benefit from multiple drug regimens. **Carbamazepine** and **valproate** are the first-line drugs in epilepsy because they cause relatively few adverse effects and seem to have least detrimental effects on cognitive function and behaviour. Some anticonvulsants, especially phenytoin, phenobarbitone and carbamazepine, are potent *liver enzyme inducers* and stimulate the metabolism of many drugs, e.g. oral contraceptives, warfarin, theophylline.

Anticonvulsant drugs, especially phenytoin, carbamazepine and valproate increase the risk of teratogenicity. Pregnant women should be offered antenatal screening and given folate supplements to reduce the risk of neural tube defects.

Carbamazepine is metabolized in the liver to carbamazepine-10,11-epoxide, an active metabolite that partly contributes to both its anticonvulsant action and neurotoxicity. In contrast to phenytoin, there is a linear increase in serum concentration with dosage. Mild neurotoxic effects are common (nausea, headache, drowsiness, diplopia and ataxia) and often determine the limit of dosage. Agranulocytosis is a rarer idiosyncratic reaction to carbamazepine.

Phenytoin is hydroxylated in the liver by a saturable enzyme system. The rate of metabolism varies greatly in different patients, and up to 20 days may be required for the serum level to stabilize after changing the dose. Therefore, the dose may be increased gradually until fits are prevented, or until signs of *cerebellar disturbance* occur (nystagmus, ataxia, dysarthria). Measurement of serum drug levels is extremely valuable because once the metabolizing enzymes are saturated, a small increase in dose may produce toxic blood levels of the drug.

Adverse effects include headache, tremor, nausea, dizziness and, with prolonged treatment, it may cause gum hypertrophy, acne, greasy skin, coarsening of the facial features and hirsutism.

Phenobarbitone is probably as effective as carbamazepine and phenytoin in the treatment of tonic–clonic and partial seizures, but it is much more sedative. Tolerance occurs with prolonged use and sudden withdrawal may precipitate status epilepticus. Side effects include *cerebellar symptoms* (e.g. sedation, ataxia, nystagmus), drowsiness in adults and hyperkinesia in children. **Primidone** is metabolized to active anticonvulsant metabolites, one of which is phenobarbitone.

Vigabatrin, gabapentin and **lamotrigine** are newer agents introduced as 'add-on' drugs in patients where epilepsy is not satisfactorily controlled by other antiepileptics. **Lamotrigine**, which can be used alone, seems to be similar to phenytoin but with fewer side effects.

DRUGS USED TO TREAT ABSENCES (PETIT MAL)

Ethosuximide is only effective in the treatment of absences and myoclonic seizures (brief jerky movements without loss of consciousness).

DRUGS EFFECTIVE IN GRAND MAL AND PETIT MAL EPILEPSY

Valproate. The advantages of valproate are its relative lack of sedative effects, its wide spectrum of activity and the mild nature of most of its adverse effects (nausea, weight gain, bleeding tendencies and transient hair loss). The main disadvantage is that occasional idiosyncratic responses cause *severe or fatal hepatic toxicity*.

Benzodiazepines. Clonazepam is a potent anticonvulsant that is effective in absences, tonic–clonic seizures and myoclonic seizures. It is very sedative and tolerance occurs with prolonged oral administration.

26 Drugs used in Parkinsonism

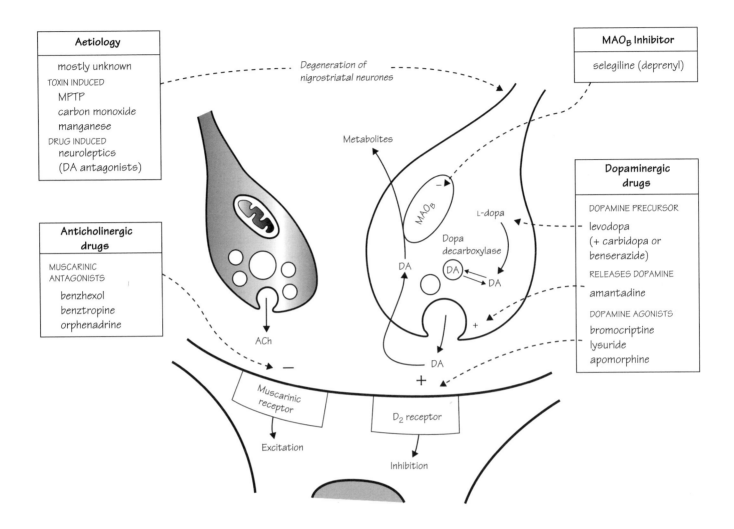

Parkinsonism is a disease of the basal ganglia and is characterized by a poverty of movement, rigidity and tremor. It is progressive and leads to increasing disability unless effective treatment is given.

In the early 1960s, analysis of brains of patients dying with Parkinsonism revealed greatly decreased levels of **dopamine** in the **basal ganglia** (caudate nucleus, putamen, globus pallidus). Parkinsonism thus became the first disease to be associated with a specific transmitter abnormality in the brain. The main pathology in Parkinsonism is extensive degeneration of the dopaminergic **nigrostriatal tract**, but the cause of the degeneration is usually unknown (top left). The cell bodies of this tract are localized in the substantia nigra in the midbrain, and it seems that frank symptoms of Parkinsonism appear only when more than 80% of these neurones have degenerated. About one-third of patients with Parkinsonism eventually develop dementia.

Replacement therapy with dopamine itself is not possible in Parkinsonism because dopamine does not pass the blood–brain barrier. However, its precursor, **levodopa** (L-dopa) does penetrate the brain, where it is decarboxylated to dopamine (right figure). Orally administered levodopa is largely metabolized outside the brain and so it is given with a selective *extracerebral decarboxylase inhibitor* (**carbidopa** or **benserazide**). This greatly decreases the effective dose by reducing peripher-

al metabolites and reduces peripheral adverse effects (*nausea, postural hypotension*). Levodopa, together with a peripheral decarboxylase inhibitor, is the mainstay of treatment. Other dopaminergic drugs used in Parkinsonism (bottom right) are directly acting **dopamine agonists** and **amantadine**, which causes dopamine release. Some of the peripheral side effects of dopaminergic drugs can be reduced with **domperidone**, a dopamine antagonist that does not penetrate the brain. Inhibition of monoamine oxidase B (MAO$_B$) with **selegiline** (top right) potentiates the actions of levodopa. Selegiline gives mild symptomatic relief when used alone but can delay the need for levodopa for a few months.

As the nigrostriatal neurones progressively degenerate in Parkinsonism, the release of (inhibitory) dopamine declines and the excitatory cholinergic interneurones in the striatum become relatively 'overactive' (left, ▭). This simple idea provides the rationale for treatment with **anticholinergic agents** (bottom left). They are most useful in controlling the tremor that is usually the presenting feature in Parkinsonism. Withdrawal of antimuscarinic drugs may worsen symptoms. Intravenous **benztropine** is used to reverse acute dystonias caused by neuroleptic drugs (Chapter 27).

AETIOLOGY

The cause of Parkinsonism is unknown and no endogenous or environmental neurotoxin has been discovered. However, the possibility that such a chemical exists has been suggested dramatically by the recent discovery in Californian drug addicts (who were trying to make pethidine) that 1-methyl-4-phenyl-1,2,3,6-tetrahydropyridine (MPTP) causes degeneration of the nigrostriatal tract and Parkinsonism. MPTP acts indirectly via a metabolite, 1-methyl-4-phenylpyridine (MPP^+), which is formed by the action of MAO_B. It is not certain how MPP^+ kills dopaminergic nerve cells, but free radicals generated during its formation by MAO_B may poison mitochondria and/or damage the cell membrane by peroxidation.

Neuroleptic drugs (Chapter 27) block dopamine receptors and often produce a Parkinsonism-like syndrome.

DOPAMINERGIC DRUGS

Levodopa with a selective extracerebral decarboxylase inhibitor is the best treatment for most patients with Parkinsonism.

Mechanism. Levodopa is the immediate precursor of dopamine and is able to penetrate the brain, where it is converted to dopamine. The site of this decarboxylation in the parkinsonian brain is uncertain, but as dopa decarboxylase is not rate limiting, there may be sufficient enzyme in the remaining dopaminergic nerve terminals. Another possibility is that the conversion occurs in noradrenergic or serotonergic terminals, because the decarboxylase activity in these neurones is not specific. In any event, the release of dopamine replaced in the brain by levodopa therapy must be very abnormal, and it is remarkable that most patients with Parkinsonism benefit, often dramatically, from its administration.

Adverse effects are frequent, and mainly result from widespread stimulation of dopamine receptors. *Nausea* and *vomiting* are caused by stimulation of the chemoreceptor trigger zone (CTZ) in the area postrema, which lies outside the blood–brain barrier. This can be reduced by the peripherally acting dopamine antagonist domperidone. *Psychiatric* side effects are the most common limiting factor in levodopa treatment and include vivid dreams, hallucinations, psychotic states and confusion. These effects are probably due to stimulation of mesolimbic or mesocortical dopamine receptors (remember overactivity in these systems is associated with schizophrenia). Postural hypotension is common but often asymptomatic. *Dyskinesias* are an important adverse effect that in the early stages of Parkinsonism usually reflect overtreatment and respond to simple dose reduction (or fractionation).

Problems with long-term treatment. After 5 years' treatment about 50% of patients will have lost ground. In some there is a gradual recurrence of parkinsonian akinesia. A second form of deterioration is the shortening of duration of action of each dose of levodopa ('*end-of-dose deterioration*'). Various dyskinesias may appear and, with time, many patients start to experience increasingly severe and rapid oscillations in mobility and dyskinesias—the '*on–off effect*. These fluctuations in response are related to the peaks and troughs of plasma levodopa levels.

It seems that progressive neuronal degeneration reduces the capacity of the striatum to buffer fluctuating levodopa levels, because continuous dopaminergic stimulation produced by the intravenous infusion of levodopa, or subcutaneous infusion of apomorphine, controls the dyskinesias. Unfortunately, this form of treatment is not generally practical, but a simpler strategy of combining oral levodopa with single injections of apomorphine given during the 'off' periods, helps many advanced fluctuating parkinsonian patients to have a more stable day.

DOPAMINE AGONISTS

Bromocriptine is a selective D_2-agonist. It is often given in combination with levodopa in the later stages of Parkinsonism in an attempt to reduce the late adverse effects of levodopa ('wearing-off' and 'on–off' phenomena). The adverse effects of bromocriptine are similar to those of levodopa (i.e. nausea, psychiatric symptoms, postural hypotension), but are more common and tend to be more severe.

Bromocriptine inhibits the release of prolactin from the pituitary and is used in the treatment of *hyperprolactinaemia*. It is also used to suppress growth hormone release in *acromegaly*, although in normal people the drug increases hormone release. The suppression of growth hormone in acromegalic people occurs because of the presence of dopamine receptors that are not expressed in normal people.

Lysuride is a D_2-agonist with similar actions to those of bromocriptine, but psychiatric side effects are more severe.

Apomorphine stimulates D_1 and D_2 dopamine receptors. It is given by subcutaneous injection in patients with advanced Parkinsonism.

DRUGS CAUSING DOPAMINE RELEASE

Amantadine has muscarinic blocking actions and probably increases dopamine release. It has modest anti-Parkinsonian effects, but tolerance soon occurs.

MAO_B INHIBITOR

Selegiline selectively inhibits MAO_B present in the brain, and for which dopamine, but not noradrenaline or serotonin, is a substrate. It reduces the metabolism of dopamine in the brain and potentiates the actions of levodopa, the dose of which can be reduced by up to one-third. Because selegiline protects animals from the effects of MPTP, it was hoped that the drug might slow the progression of Parkinsonism in patients. Unfortunately it does not.

ANTICHOLINERGIC AGENTS

Muscarinic antagonists produce a modest improvement in the early stages of Parkinsonism, but the akinesia that is responsible for most of the functional disability responds least well. Furthermore, adverse effects are common and include dry mouth, urinary retention and constipation. More seriously, anticholinergics can affect memory and concentration and precipitate an organic confusional state with visual hallucinations, especially in elderly or dementing patients.

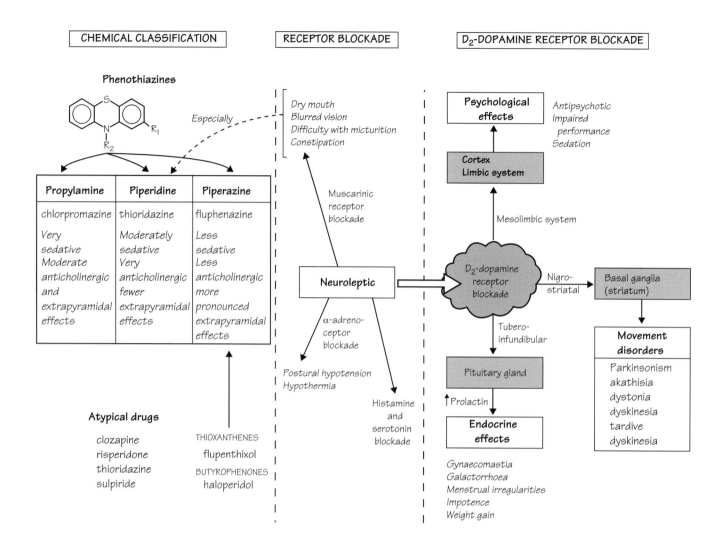

Schizophrenia is a syndrome characterized by specific psychological manifestations. These include auditory hallucinations, delusions, thought disorders and behavioural disturbances. Recent evidence suggests that schizophrenia is caused by developmental abnormalities involving the medial temporal lobe (parahippocampal gyrus, hippocampus and amygdala), temporal, and frontal lobe cortex. Schizophrenia can be a genetically determined illness but there is also evidence implicating intrauterine events and obstetric complications. Neuroleptic drugs control many of the symptoms of schizophrenia. They have most effect on the positive symptoms such as hallucinations and delusion. Negative symptoms such as social withdrawal and emotional apathy are less affected by neuroleptic drugs. About 30% of patients show only limited improvement, and 7% show no improvement even with prolonged treatment. The neuroleptics are all **antagonists at dopamine receptors**, suggesting that schizophrenia is associated with increased activity in the dopaminergic *mesolimbic* and/or *mesocortical pathway* (top right). In agreement with this idea, amphetamine (which causes noradrenaline and dopamine release) can produce a psychotic state in normal subjects, indistinguishable from paranoid schizophrenia. Neuroleptic drugs require several weeks to control the symptoms of schizophrenia and most patients will require maintenance treatment for many years. Relapses are common even in drug-maintained patients and more than two-thirds of patients relapse within a year if they stop drug treatment.

Unfortunately, neuroleptics also block dopamine receptors in the basal ganglia (striatum) and this frequently results in distressing and disabling **movement disorders** (extrapyramidal effects) (right). These include Parkinsonism and acute dystonic reactions (which may require treatment with anticholinergic drugs), akathisia (motor restlessness) and tardive dyskinesia (orofacial and trunk movements), which may be irreversible. It is not known what causes tardive dyskinesia, but because it may be made worse by removing the drug, it has been suggested that the striatal dopamine receptors become supersensitive. Some **'atypical' drugs** (bottom left) are free or relatively free of extrapyramidal side effects at low doses, but only clozapine never causes them.

In the pituitary gland, dopamine acting on D_2-dopamine receptors inhibits prolactin release. This effect is blocked by neuroleptics and the resulting increase in prolactin release often causes **endocrine side effects** (bottom right).

Neuroleptics have muscarinic receptor and α-adrenoceptor blocking actions and cause **autonomic side effects** (middle), including postural hypotension, dry mouth and constipation. The potency of individual drugs in blocking autonomic receptors, and therefore their predominant peripheral side effects, depends on the **chemical class** to which they belong (left).

DOPAMINE RECEPTORS

Dopamine receptors were originally subdivided into two types (D_1 and D_2). Currently there are five cloned dopamine receptors that fall into these two classes. The D_1-like receptors include D_1 and D_5, whilst the D_2-like receptors include D_2, D_3 and D_4. The dopamine receptors all display the seven transmembrane-spanning domains characteristic of G-protein-linked receptors and are linked to adenylyl cyclase stimulation (D_1) or inhibition (D_2).

D_1-like dopamine receptors (subtypes D_1, D_5) are involved mainly in postsynaptic inhibition. Most neuroleptic drugs block D_1-receptors but this action does not correlate with their antipsychotic activity. In particular, the *butyrophenones* are potent neuroleptics, but are weak D_1-receptor antagonists.

D_2-like dopamine receptors (subtypes D_2, D_3, D_4) are involved in presynaptic and postsynaptic inhibition. Most of the known functions of dopamine seem to involve D_2-like receptors. The affinity of neuroleptic drugs for the D_2-receptor correlates closely with their antipsychotic potency and this provides circumstantial evidence that schizophrenia is somehow linked to 'overactivity' in a central dopaminergic pathway and that D_2-receptors are involved. D_2- receptors (and also D_3- and D_4-receptors) occur in the limbic system, which is concerned with mood and emotional stability. Because there are high densities of D_2-receptors in the areas of the caudate nucleus that receive fibres from the nigrostriatal tract, neuroleptics often cause movement disorders. It is not known whether the antipsychotic effects of neuroleptic drugs involve blockade of D_3-receptors as well as D_2-receptors. **Clozapine** is unique in having a particularly high affinity for the D_4-receptors but a low affinity for D_2-receptors.

Mechanism of action of neuroleptics. It is not known how neuroleptic drugs reduce the severity of the symptoms in schizophrenia. Since all antipsychotic drugs are dopamine antagonists, it is assumed that schizophrenia is associated with 'overactivity' in the mesolimbic/mesocortical pathways. However, it has proved difficult to find convincing changes in the dopaminergic system of patients with schizophrenia.

CHEMICAL CLASSIFICATION

Drugs with a wide variety of structures have antipsychotic activity, but they all have the ability to block dopamine receptors in common.

Phenothiazines are subdivided according to the type of side-chain attached to the N-atom of the phenothiazine ring.
1 Propylamine side-chain. Phenothiazines with an aliphatic side-chain have relatively low potency and produce nearly all of the side effects shown in the figure. **Chlorpromazine** was the first phenothiazine used in schizophrenia and is widely used, although it produces more adverse effects than newer drugs. It is very sedative and is particularly useful in treating violent patients. Adverse effects include sensitivity reactions such as agranulocytosis, haemolytic anaemia, rashes, cholestatic jaundice and photosensitization.
2 Piperidine side-chain. The main drug in this group is **thiori-**dazine. The advantage of this drug, use of which is favoured in the elderly, is that it is relatively rarely associated with movement disorders and does not cause troublesome hangover drowsiness. Anticholinergic activity is marked and it may cause sexual dysfunction, including retrograde ejaculation. Rarely, high doses may cause retinal degeneration.
3 Piperazine side-chain. Drugs in this group include **fluphenazine, perphenazine** and **trifluoperazine.** They are less sedative and less anticholinergic than chlorpromazine, but are particularly likely to cause movement disorders, especially in the elderly, for whom thioridazine is preferred.

Other chemical classes

Butyrophenones. **Haloperidol** has little anticholinergic action and is less sedative and hypotensive than chlorpromazine. However, there is a high incidence of movement disorders.

Atypical drugs (clozapine, risperidone, thioridazine, sulpiride) are so called because they are associated with a lower incidence of movement disorders but the reason for this is not known. **Clozapine** is regarded by some as the only truly atypical neuroleptic, because it is sometimes effective in patients refractory to other neuroleptic drugs and almost never causes movement disorders. The drug is restricted to this group of refractory patients because it causes neutropenia in about 3% and potentially fatal agranulocytosis in about 1% of patients (blood samples are required regularly to monitor white cells). Clozapine may be atypical because at clinically effective doses it blocks D_4-receptors (present mainly in limbic areas) with relatively little effect on striatal D_2-receptors. However, clozapine blocks many other receptors (centre figure) including muscarinic and $5HT_2$ receptors. Since anticholinergic drugs prevent neuroleptic-induced movement disorders, it is possible that blockade of muscarinic receptors accounts for the atypical action of clozapine, but **thioridazine**, which also has a high affinity for muscarinic receptors, may cause extrapyramidal effects at higher doses. Another suggestion is that the atypical action of clozapine is due to its potent block of $5HT_2$ receptors. However, this is pure speculation and ritanserin (a $5HT_2$ antagonist) has no effect on hallucinations and delusions. **Risperidone** is a newer drug that is non-sedative and lacks anticholinergic and α-blocking actions. It blocks $5HT_2$ receptors but is a more potent antagonist than clozapine at D_2-receptors. At low doses, it does not cause extrapyramidal effects but this advantage is lost with higher doses. **Sulpiride** is a very specific D_2-blocker that is widely used because it has a low liability for extrapyramidal effects and, although quite sedating, can be well tolerated. It has been suggested that sulpiride has a higher affinity for mesolimbic D_2-receptors than striatal D_2-receptors.

DEPOT PREPARATIONS

Schizophrenic patients are increasingly being 'returned to the community'. This has led to an increased use of long-acting depot injections for maintenance therapy. Oily injections of the decanoate derivatives of **flupenthixol, haloperidol** and **fluphenazine** may be given at intervals of 1–4 weeks, but these preparations increase the incidence of movement disorders.

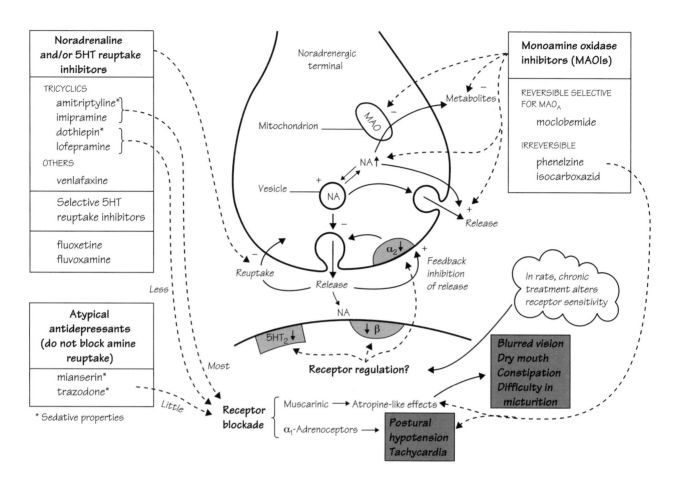

Affective disorders are characterized by a disturbance of mood associated with alterations in behaviour, energy, appetite, sleep and weight. The extremes range from intense excitement and elation (**mania**) to severe **depressive states**. In depression, which is much more common than mania, a person becomes persistently sad and unhappy. Depression is common, and although it can cause people to kill themselves, in general the prognosis is good.

Most of the drugs used in the treatment of depression inhibit the reuptake of noradrenaline (NA) and/or serotonin (5HT) (top left). The **tricyclics** are older drugs with proven efficacy but are often sedative and have autonomic side effects (▇) that may limit their use. The tricyclics are the most dangerous in overdosage, mainly because of cardiotoxicity, but convulsions are common. **Selective serotonin reuptake inhibitors** (SSRIs) are newer drugs that have a wide margin of safety and a different spectrum of side effects (mainly gastrointestinal). **Monoamine oxidase inhibitors** (MAOIs) (top right) have been used less often because of dangerous interactions with some foods and drugs. However, the recent introduction of reversible inhibitors of MAO type A (RIMAs) (top right) has led to some increase in the use of this type of drug.

Some 'atypical' antidepressants are not MAOIs and do not inhibit amine uptake (bottom left). All antidepressants may provoke seizures and no particular drug is safe for the depressed epileptic patient. A striking characteristic of antidepressant treatment with drugs is that the benefit does not become apparent for 2–3 weeks. The reason for this is unknown, but may be related to gradual changes in the sensitivity of central 5HT and/or adrenoceptors (▇). About 70% of patients respond satisfactorily to treatment with antidepressant drugs, but in severe or refractory cases of depression, electroconvulsive therapy (ECT) may be required in addition. In patients who fail to respond to single drugs and/or ECT, some psychiatrists combine tricyclics with MAOIs or lithium but dangerous interactions can occur with these drug combinations. Following a response, antidepressant drugs should be continued for 4–6 months because this reduces the incidence of relapse. Abrupt withdrawal of antidepressant drugs, especially MAOIs, may cause nausea, vomiting, panic, anxiety and motor restlessness.

The cause of depression and the mechanisms of action of antidepressants are unknown. The **monoamine theory** was based on the idea that depression resulted from a decrease in the activity of central noradrenergic and/or serotonergic systems. There are serious problems with this theory, but it has not been replaced with a better one. More recently, interest has focused on the effects of antidepressant treatment on **receptor regulation** in the brain.

In *mania* and in *bipolar affective disorders* (where mania alternates with depression) **lithium** has a mood-stabilizing action. Lithium salts have a low therapeutic:toxic ratio and adverse effects are common. **Carbamazepine** also has mood-stabilizing properties and can be used in patients who do not respond to, or are unable to take, lithium.

Monoamine theory of depression. *Reserpine*, which depletes the brain of NA and serotonin, often causes depression. In contrast, the *tricyclics* and related compounds block the reuptake of NA and/or serotonin and the MAOIs increase their concentration in the brain. Both of these actions increase the amounts of NA and/or serotonin available in the synaptic cleft. These drug effects suggest that depression might be associated with a decrease in brain NA and/or serotonin function. Much effort has gone into trying to find the expected defects in central noradrenergic and serotonergic systems in depressed patients, but these studies have not produced consistent results. There are several problems with the monoamine theory of depression. In particular, it is difficult to understand why the tricyclic drugs rapidly block NA/serotonin uptake but require weeks of administration to achieve an antidepressant effect. Also, some drugs are antidepressant but do not affect amine uptake (e.g. mianserin, trazodone), whilst cocaine blocks uptake but is not antidepressant.

Receptor regulation. Chronic adminstration of antidepressants to rodents gradually decreases the sensitivity of central $5HT_2$ receptors, β_1- and α_2-adrenoceptors (downregulation). Whether similar changes in receptor sensitivity underlie the antidepressant action of drugs in humans is unknown, but chronic antidepressant treatment has been shown to lower the sensitivity of clonidine (an α_2-adrenoceptor agonist).

DRUGS THAT INHIBIT AMINE UPTAKE

The term 'tricyclic drug' originally referred to compounds based on the dibenzazepine (e.g. **imipramine**) and dibenzocyclohepadiene (e.g. **amitriptyline**) ring structures. This widely used term is now misleading because many second-generation antidepressants with similar pharmacological properties to the original tricyclics, possess one, two or four rings.

No individual tricyclic drug has superior antidepressant activity and the choice of drug is determined by the most acceptable or desired side effects. Thus, drugs with sedative actions such as **amitriptyline** and **dothiepin** are more suitable for agitated and anxious patients and, if given at bedtime, will also act as a hypnotic. The tricyclics resemble the phenothiazines in structure and have similar blocking actions at cholinergic *muscarinic receptors*, *α-adrenoreceptors* and *histamine receptors*. These actions frequently cause dry mouth, blurred vision, constipation, urinary retention, tachycardia and postural hypotension. In overdosage, the anticholinergic activity and a quinidine-like action of the tricyclics on the heart may cause arrhythmias and sudden death. *They are contraindicated in heart disease.*

The SSRIs do not have the troublesome autonomic side effects or appetite-stimulating effects of the tricyclics, but do have different ones, the commonest being nausea, vomiting, diarrhoea and constipation. The SSRIs are now generally accepted as first-line drugs, especially in patients with cardiovascular disease, or in whom any sedation must be avoided, or for those who cannot tolerate the anticholinergic effects of the tricyclics. **Venlafaxine** is a new drug that inhibits the reuptake of both 5HT and noradrenaline but lacks the receptor blocking actions of the tricyclics.Its adverse effects resemble those of the SSRIs.

ATYPICAL ANTIDEPRESSANTS

These drugs have little or no activity on amine uptake. They generally cause fewer autonomic side effects and because they are less car-diotoxic they are less dangerous in overdosage. **Mianserin** and **trazodone** are sedative antidepressants. Mianserin has α_2-adrenoceptor blocking activity and by blocking inhibitory α_2-autoreceptors on central noradrenergic nerve endings, it may increase the amount of NA in the synaptic cleft. Mianserin may cause agranulocytosis and aplastic anaemia (particularly in the elderly).

MAOIs

The older MAOIs (e.g. **phenelzine**) are irreversible non-selective inhibitors of MAO and appear to be most useful in atypical depression and phobic anxiety states. Their usefulness is limited by adverse effects (postural hypotension, dizziness, anticholinergic effects and liver damage) and by interactions with sympathomimetic amines (e.g. *ephedrine*, often present in cough mixtures and decongestive preparations), or foods containing *tyramine* (e.g. cheese, game, alcoholic drinks) which may result in severe hypertension. Ingested tyramine is normally metabolized by MAO in the gut wall and liver, but when the enzyme is inhibited, tyramine reaches the circulation and causes the release of NA from sympathetic nerve endings (indirect sympathomimetic action). MAOIs are not specific and reduce the metabolism of barbiturates, opioid analgesics and alcohol. Pethidine is especially dangerous in patients taking MAOIs, causing (by an unknown mechanism) hyperpyrexia, hypotension and coma. **Moclobemide** is a reversible inhibitor that selectively inhibits monoamine oxidase A (cf. selegiline, Chapter 26). It is well tolerated, the main side effects being insomnia and nausea. Moclobemide interacts with the same drugs as other MAOIs but because it is reversible the effects of the interaction rapidly diminish when the drug is discontinued. Moclobemide is a second-line drug used in depression after tricyclics and SSRIs.

Lithium is used for prophylaxis in *manic/depressive* illness. It is also used in the treatment of *acute mania*, but, because it may take several days for the antimanic effect to develop, an antipsychotic drug is usually preferred for acutely disturbed patients. Lithium is used as an **antidepressant** in combination with tricyclics in refractory patients.

Lithium is rapidly absorbed from the gut. The therapeutic and toxic doses are similar and serum lithium concentrations must be measured regularly (therapeutic range 0.4–1.0 mM). Adverse effects include nausea, vomiting, anorexia, diarrhoea, tremor of the hands, polydipsia and polyuria (a few patients develop nephrogenic diabetes insipidus), hypothyroidism and weight gain. Signs of *lithium toxicity* include drowsiness, ataxia and confusion, and at serum levels above 2–3 mM, life-threatening seizures and coma may occur.

Mechanism of action. This is unknown, but much current interest is focused on interactions with second-messenger systems. In particular, lithium at concentrations of less than 1 mM blocks the phosphatidylinositol (PI) pathway at the point where inositol-1-phosphate is hydrolysed to inositol. This causes depletion of membrane PIP_2 (see Chapter 1) and may reduce the actions of transmitters acting at receptors which involve inositol trisphosphate/diacylglycerol ($InsP_3$/DG) as their second messengers.

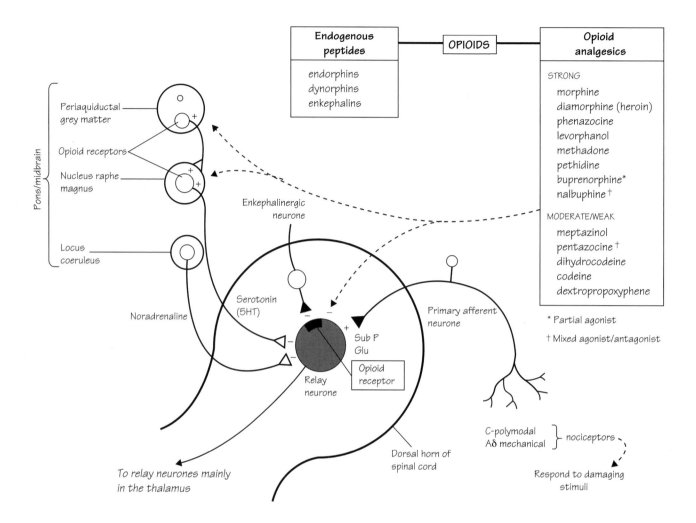

Endogenous peptides	OPIOIDS	Opioid analgesics
endorphins		STRONG
dynorphins		morphine
enkephalins		diamorphine (heroin)

Pain receptors, when stimulated by noxious stimuli, initiate firing in primary afferent fibres which synapse in lamina I and II of the dorsal horn of the spinal cord. The relay neurones ( ) in the dorsal horn transmit pain information to the sensory cortex via neurones in the thalamus. Little is known about the transmitter substances utilized in the ascending pain pathways, but some primary afferent fibres are thought to release peptides (e.g. substance P, calcitonin gene-related peptides) (lower figure, shaded).

The activity of the dorsal horn relay neurones is modulated by several *inhibitory inputs*. These include local interneurones, which release **opioid peptides** (e.g. met-enkephalin), and descending *noradrenergic* and *serotonergic* fibres, which originate in the brainstem (top left) and are themselves activated by *opioid peptides*. Thus, opioid peptide release in both the brainstem and the spinal cord can *reduce* the activity of the dorsal horn relay neurones and can cause analgesia. How the different inhibitory mechanisms are normally controlled is unknown, but the effects of opioid peptides are mediated by specific **opioid receptors.**

Opioid analgesics (right) are drugs that mimic endogenous opioid peptides by causing a prolonged activation of opioid receptors (usually μ-receptors). This produces analgesia, respiratory depression, euphoria and sedation. Opioids often cause nausea and vomiting and anti-emetics

may be required. Effects on the nerve plexuses in the gut, which also possess opioid peptides and receptors, causes constipation, and laxatives are usually required (Chapter 13). Continuous treatment with opioid analgesics results in **tolerance** and **dependence** in addicts. However, in terminally ill patients a steady increase in morphine dosage is not automatic, and where it does occur is more likely to result from progressively increasing pain rather than tolerance. Similarly, in the clinical context, dependence is unimportant. *Unfortunately, overcaution in the use of opioid analgesics frequently results in unnecessarily poor pain control in patients.*

Some analgesics, such as **codeine**, are less potent than morphine and cannot be given in equianalgesic doses because of the onset of adverse effects. As a result of this restriction in dosage, they are less likely, in practice, to produce respiratory depression and dependence. They are useful in controlling mild to moderate pain.

Naloxone is a specific antagonist at opioid receptors and reverses respiratory depression caused by morphine-like drugs. It also precipitates a withdrawal syndrome when dependence has occurred. Electroacupuncture analgesia, transcutaneous nerve stimulation-induced analgesia and placebo effects can sometimes be partially blocked by naloxone, suggesting the involvement of the endogenous opioid peptides.

Opioids are defined as compounds with effects that are antagonized by naloxone. There are three families of **opioid peptides** which are derived from large precursor molecules, encoded for by separate genes. *Pro-opiomelanocortin* (POMC) gives rise to the opioid peptide β-endorphin and a number of other non-opioid peptides, including adrenocorticotrophic hormone (ACTH). *Proenkephalin* gives rise to leu-enkephalin and met-enkephalin. *Prodynorphin* gives rise to a number of opioid peptides which contain leu-enkephalin at their amino terminal (e.g. dynorphin A). The peptides derived from each of these three precursor molecules have a distinct anatomical distribution in the central nervous system and have varying affinity for the different types of opioid receptors. The precise function of these opioid peptides in the brain and elsewhere is still unclear.

Opioid receptors are widely distributed throughout the central nervous system and have been classified into three main types. The μ-receptors are most highly concentrated in brain areas involved in nociception and are the receptors with which most opioid analgesics interact to produce analgesia. The δ- and κ-receptors display selectivity for the enkephalins and the dynorphins, respectively. Activation of κ-receptors also produces analgesia but in contrast to μ-agonists (e.g. **morphine**), which cause euphoria, κ-agonists (e.g. **pentazocine, nalbuphine**) are associated with dysphoria. Some opioid analgesics (e.g. *pentazocine*) produce stimulant and psychotomimetic effects by acting on σ-receptors. (Phencyclidine, a psychotomimetic drug, binds to these receptors.) Since these effects are not blocked by naloxone, σ-receptors are not opioid receptors. The opioid peptides have inhibitory actions on synapses in the central nervous system and gut. Activation of μ- and δ-receptors causes hyperpolarization of neurones by activating K^+ channels by a process involving a G-protein. Activation of κ-receptors inhibits membrane Ca^{2+} channels.

STRONG OPIOID ANALGESICS

These are used particularly in the treatment of dull, poorly localized (visceral) pain. Somatic pain is sharply defined and may be relieved by a weak opioid analgesic or by a non-steroidal anti-inflammatory drug (NSAID) (Chapter 32). **Parenteral morphine** is widely used to treat severe pain and **oral morphine** is the drug of choice in terminal care.

Morphine and other opioid analgesics produce a range of central effects that include analgesia, euphoria, sedation, respiratory depression, depression of the vasomotor centre (causing postural hypotension), miosis because of IIIrd nerve nucleus stimulation (except pethidine which has weak atropine-like activity), and nausea and vomiting due to stimulation of the chemoreceptor trigger zone. They also cause cough suppression, but this is not correlated with their opioid activity. Peripheral effects which include constipation, biliary spasm and constriction of the sphincter of Oddi may occur. Morphine may cause histamine release with vasodilatation and itching. Morphine is metabolized in the liver by conjugation with glucuronic acid to form morphine-3-glucuronide, which is inactive, and morphine-6-glucuronide, which is a more potent analgesic than morphine itself, especially when given intrathecally.

Tolerance (i.e. a decreased responsiveness) to many of the effects of opioid analgesics occurs with continuous administration. Miosis and constipation are effects to which little tolerance develops.

Dependence. Both physical and psychological dependence on opioid analgesics gradually develops and sudden termination of drug administration precipitates a withdrawal syndrome (Chapter 31).

Diamorphine (heroin, diacetylmorphine) is twice as potent as morphine, but is rapidly metabolized to 6-acetylmorphine (which is active) and more slowly to morphine. It causes more euphoria but relatively less nausea, constipation and hypotension than morphine.

Methadone is well absorbed orally and has a long duration of action. It is used orally for maintenance treatment of heroin or morphine addicts in whom it prevents the 'buzz' of intravenous drugs (see also Chapter 31).

Pethidine is similar to morphine but shorter acting. Equianalgesic doses depress respiration equally, but it is a poor antitussive and is less constipating. Pethidine is more lipid soluble than morphine, giving it a rapid onset of action. Pethidine is metabolized in the liver and at high doses norpethidine can accumulate; this has excitatory actions (dilated pupil, convulsions). Pethidine interacts seriously with MAOIs (Chapter 28) causing delirium, hyperpyrexia and convulsions or respiratory depression.

Buprenorphine is a partial agonist at μ-receptors. It is very lipid soluble and is an effective analgesic following sublingual administration. It has a much longer duration of action than morphine but may cause prolonged vomiting. Respiratory depression, if it occurs, is difficult to reverse with naloxone, because buprenorphine dissociates very slowly from the receptors.

Nalbuphine is a κ-agonist and a μ-antagonist that is equipotent with morphine in producing analgesia and respiratory depression, but produces less nausea and vomiting. At higher doses it causes dysphoria.

WEAK OPIOID ANALGESICS

Weak opioid analgesics are used in 'mild-to-moderate' pain. They may cause dependence and are subject to abuse. However, they are less attractive to addicts because they do not give a good 'buzz'.

Pentazocine is an unpleasant weak analgesic orally, but when given by injection its efficacy is somewhere between that of morphine and codeine. It is an agonist at κ- and σ-receptors, but an antagonist at μ-receptors. It is less likely to cause dependence. This may be partly due to the frequency with which it causes hallucinations, bad dreams and thought disorders due to activation of σ-receptors.

Codeine (methylmorphine) is well absorbed orally but has a very low affinity for opioid receptors. About 10% of the drug is demethylated in the liver to morphine, which is responsible for the analgesic effects of codeine. Side effects (constipation, vomiting, sedation) limit the possible dosage to levels that produce much less analgesia than morphine. Codeine is also used as an antitussive and antidiarrhoeal agent.

Dextropropoxyphene is about half as potent as codeine, but has similar actions at equianalgesic doses. It is often give in fixed combinations with aspirin or paracetamol (e.g. co-proxamol) but there is little evidence that such combinations are more effective than the NSAID alone. Combinations with paracetamol are dangerous in overdose because the dextropropoxyphene causes respiratory depression and acute heart failure, whilst the paracetamol is hepatotoxic.

30 Drugs used in nausea and vertigo (anti-emetics)

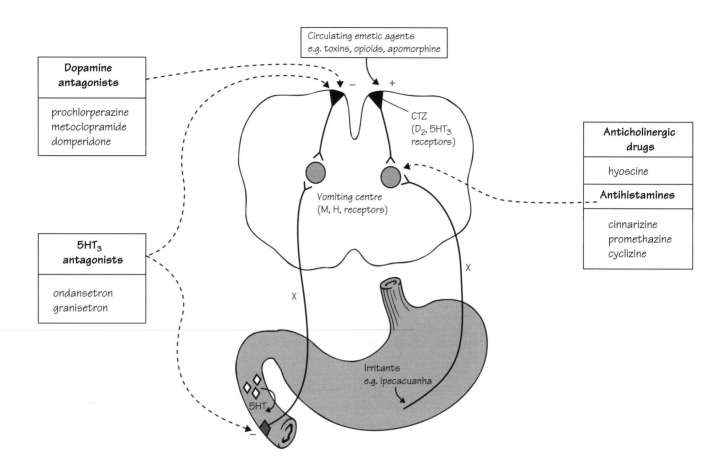

Nausea and vomiting has many causes, including drugs (e.g. cytotoxic agents, opioids, anaesthetics, digoxin), vestibular disease, provocative movement (e.g. sea-sickness), migraine, pregnancy. Vomiting is much easier to prevent than to stop once it has started. Therefore, if possible, anti-emetics should be given well before the emetic stimulus is expected. Anti-emetics should not be given before the diagnosis is known because identification of the underlying cause may be delayed.

Emesis is co-ordinated by the **vomiting centre** (⬤) in the medulla (upper figure). An important source of stimulation of the vomiting centre is the **chemoreceptor trigger zone** (CTZ) (▼) in the area postrema. Because the CTZ is not protected by the blood–brain barrier (it is part of the circumventricular system) it can be stimulated by circulating toxins or drugs (top). The CTZ possesses many dopamine (D_2) receptors, which explains why dopaminergic drugs used in the treatment of Parkinson's disease frequently cause nausea and vomiting. On the other hand, **dopamine receptor antagonists** are **anti-emetics** (upper left) and are used to reduce nausea and vomiting associated with the administration of emetogenic drugs (e.g. many cytotoxic anticancer agents).

Recently, **$5HT_3$ antagonists** (e.g. ondansetron, left lower) have been found to be effective antiemetics, and because they have fewer unwanted actions they are increasingly being used to prevent or reduce the nausea and vomiting associated with cancer chemotherapy and general anaesthesia. It is uncertain how $5HT_3$ antagonists produce their antiemetic effects. There is a high concentration of $5HT_3$ receptors in the CTZ, but a peripheral action may also be important. Many cytotoxic drugs (and X-radiation) cause the release of 5HT from enterochromaffin cells (◇) in the gut, and this activates $5HT_3$ receptors on vagal sensory fibres (◆) (lower figure). Stimulation of sensory fibres in the stomach by irritants (e.g. ipecacuanha, bacterial toxins) causes 'reflex' nausea and vomiting.

Dopamine antagonists and $5HT_3$ antagonists are ineffective in reducing the nausea and vomiting of **motion sickness**. **Anticholinergic drugs** or **antihistamines** (right), which act directly on the vomiting centre, may be effective, although side effects are common. Vertigo and vomiting associated with **vestibular disease** are treated with **antihistamines** (e.g. promazine, cinnarizine), **phenothiazines** or **betahistine**.

The **vomiting centre** is in the lateral reticular formation of the medulla at the level of the olivary nuclei. It receives afferents from the following.

1 *Limbic cortex.* These presumably account for the nausea associated with unpleasant odours and sights. Cortical afferents are also involved in the conditioned vomiting reflex that may occur when patients see or smell the cytotoxic drugs they are about to receive.

2 The *CTZ*.

3 *Nucleus solitarius.* These complete the arc for the gag reflex (i.e. the reflex caused by poking a finger in the mouth).

4 *Spinal cord* (spinoreticular fibres). These are involved in the nausea that accompanies physical injury.

5 *Vestibular system.* These are involved in the nausea and vomiting associated with vestibular disease and motion sickness.

The transmitters involved in the pathways concerned with emesis are not fully known. However, the CTZ is rich in dopamine-D_2 and $5HT_3$ receptors. Cholinergic and histaminergic synapses are involved in transmission from the vestibular apparatus to the vomiting centre.

The vomiting centre projects to the vagus nerve and to the spinal motor neurones supplying the abdominal muscles. It is responsible for co-ordinating the complex events underlying emesis. Reverse peristalsis transfers the contents of the upper intestine into the stomach. The glottis closes, the breath is held, and oesophagus and gastric sphincter relax, and finally the abdominal muscles contract, ejecting the gastric contents.

Drug-induced vomiting. Cytotoxic drugs vary in their emetic potential, but some, e.g. cisplatin, cause severe vomiting in most patients. The emetic action of these drugs seems to involve the CTZ, and the dopamine antagonists are often effective anti-emetics. **Prochlorperazine** is phenothiazine that has been widely used as an anti-emetic. It is less sedative than chlorpromazine but may cause severe dystonic reactions (like all typical neuroleptics, Chapter 27). **Metoclopramide** is a D_2-antagonist but also has a prokinetic action on the gut and increases the absorption of many drugs (Chapter 13). This can be an advantage, e.g. in migraine, where the absorption of analgesics is enhanced. Adverse effects are usually mild but severe dystonic reactions may occur (more commonly in the young and in females). **Domperidone** is similar to metoclopramide but does not pass the blood–brain barrier and rarely causes sedation or extrapyramidal effects. The $5HT_3$ antagonists, e.g. **ondansetron**, lack the adverse effects of dopamine antagonists but may cause constipation or headaches. It has been shown in clinical trials that the severe vomiting caused by highly emetic cytotoxic drugs is controlled better by combinations of intravenous anti-emetic drugs, e.g. **metoclopramide** and **dexamethasone**. A combination of **ondansetron** and **dexamethasone** will prevent cisplatin-induced emesis in most patients. It is not known why dexamethasone is anti-emetic.

Motion sickness is very common and includes sea-sickness, air-sickness, etc. It is characterized by pallor, cold sweating, nausea and vomiting. The symptoms and signs develop relatively gradually but eventually culminate in vomiting or retching, after which there is often a temporary lessening of malaise. Continued exposure to the provocative motion (e.g. of a ship) leads to increasing protective adaptation and after 4 days most people are symptom free. Motion sickness is believed to be a response to conflicting sensory information (i.e. signals from the eye and vestibular system do not agree). Little is known about the neural mechanisms involved in motion sickness but it does not occur following labyrinthectomy or ablation of the vestibular cerebellum.

Procedures that reduce vestibular/visual conflict may help. For example, avoid head movements, and if on the deck of a ship one should fixate on the horizon, but if enclosed in a cabin it is better to close one's eyes. **Hyoscine** is one of the most effective agents that reduce the incidence of motion sickness. It is a muscarinic receptor antagonist and frequently causes drowsiness, dry mouth and blurred vision. **Cinnarizine** is an antihistamine. It has an efficacy similar to that of hyoscine but produces fewer side effects. It must be taken 2 hours before exposure to provocative stimulation.

Vestibular disease. The labyrinths generate a continuous input to the brainstem. Any pathological process that alters the balance of this *tonus* may cause dizziness (anything from lightness in the head to the inability to stand or walk). The major symptom is *vertigo*, which is a false sense of rotary movement, associated with sympathetic overactivity, nausea and vomiting.

Acute labyrinthitis often presents abruptly as vertigo with nausea and vomiting. It is frequently regarded as a viral or postviral syndrome. **Menières disease** results from increased pressure in the membranous labyrinth. Attacks of severe vertigo associated with nausea, vomiting, deafness and tinnitus occur several times, followed by long periods of remission. Between attacks, the deafness and tinnitus persist and gradually worsen. *Anti-emetics* used in labyrinth disease include **antihistamines** (**cinnarizine, cyclizine**) and **phenothiazines** (**promazine, prochlorperazine**). **Betahistine** is a drug used specifically in Menières disease because it is supposed to act by reducing endolymphatic pressure.

Pregnancy. Anti-emetics should only be used for intractable vomiting because of possible (but undefined) risk to the foetus. Limited evidence suggests that **promethazine** is safe.

31 Drug misuse and dependence

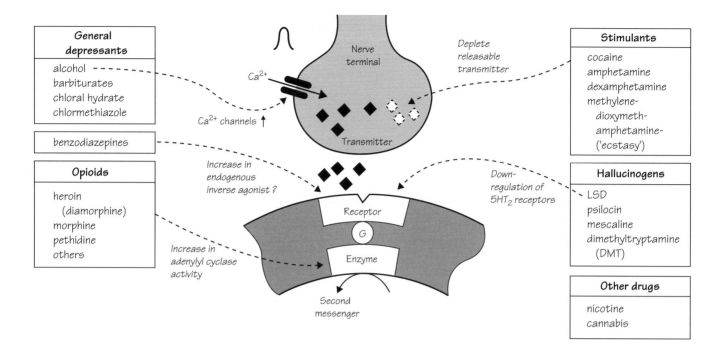

The relationship between drugs that act on the mind and society is one of an uneasy and changing coexistence. For example, there is much popular concern today about the illicit use of opioids, but in the nineteenth century, laudenum, an alcoholic solution of opium, was a popular and readily available home medication. Society now accepts only **alcohol** and **nicotine** (tobacco) as legal psychoactive drugs, although their misuse is responsible for considerable morbidity and mortality. Smoking is by far the commonest drug dependency in the UK and causes 100 000 deaths each year in Britain; it is the biggest cause of avoidable premature death.

The term **drug misuse** is applied to any drug-taking which harms or threatens to harm the physical or mental health of an individual, or other individuals, or which is illegal. Thus, drug misuse includes *alcohol* and *nicotine* and the deleterious over-prescription of medicines (e.g. **benzodiazepines, stimulants**), as well as the more obvious taking of illicit drugs.

Drug dependence is a term used when a person has a compulsion to take a drug in order to experience its psychic effects, and sometimes to avoid the discomfort of withdrawal symptoms.

The likelihood of drug misuse leading to dependence depends on many factors, including the *type of drug*, the *route of administration*, the *pattern of drug-taking* and the *individual*. Rapid delivery systems (i.e. intravenous injection, smoking cocaine or heroin) increase the dependence potential. Intravenous injections have attendant dangers of infection (acquired immune deficiency syndrome (AIDS), hepatitis, septicaemia, etc.).

Drug dependence is often associated with **tolerance**, a phenomenon that may occur with chronic adminstration of a drug. It is characterized by the necessity to progressively increase the dose of the drug to produce its original effect. Tolerance may be due, in part, to increased metabolism of the drug (pharmacokinetic tolerance), but it is mainly caused by neuroadaptive changes in the brain.

The mechanisms underlying drug dependence and tolerance are poorly understood. In general, chronic drug administration induces homeostatic adaptive changes in the brain that operate in a manner to oppose the action of the drug. Withdrawal of the drug causes a rebound in central excitability. Thus, the withdrawal of depressants (e.g. alcohol, barbiturates) may result in convulsions, whilst the withdrawal of excitatory drugs (e.g. amphetamine) results in depression.

Many neuroadaptive changes in the brain have been described following chronic drug administration. They include an increase in Ca^{2+} channels (top left), depletion of transmitter (top right), receptor downregulation (middle right), changes in second messenger (bottom left) and the synthesis of an inverse agonist (middle left).

The brain circuits involved in drug dependence are not known. However, there is evidence from animal experiments that one important circuit is the dopaminergic pathway from the ventral tegmental area that projects to the nucleus accumbens and prefrontal cortex. By the use of microdialysis techniques which can measure transmitter release from discrete brain areas, it has been shown that many drugs of dependence (e.g. stimulants, opioids, nicotine, alcohol) increase dopamine release in the nucleus accumbens and/or the frontal cortex. Some (e.g. amphetamine, cocaine) act on nerve terminals, whilst opioids increase dopamine release by inhibiting GABAergic input onto the dopaminergic neurones. Animals will self-administer cocaine and opioids into the nucleus accumbens and the 'pleasure' this causes reinforces the self-administration. A similar reward system may be involved in human drug dependence.

Central stimulants

Amphetamine-like drugs given orally decrease appetite, give a sense of increased energy and well-being and enhance physical performance. They also have peripheral sympathomimetic effects (e.g. hypertension, tachycardia) and cause insomnia. Amphetamine-like drugs cause dopamine and noradrenaline release from nerve terminals, but their behavioural effects are due mainly to dopamine release. **Cocaine** blocks the reuptake of dopamine into nerve terminals and has very similar effects to amphetamine.

Central stimulants have few indications. They *should not be used as appetite suppressants* in the treatment of obesity, because they do not improve the long-term outlook and often result in dependence.

Cocaine hydrochloride is usually 'snorted' up the nose, but the free base ('crack'), which is more volatile, can be smoked, whereupon it is rapidly absorbed through the lungs and produces a sudden, brief, but overwhelming, sense of euphoria ('rush'). A similar 'rush' is produced by intravenous amphetamine and addicts cannot distinguish between them. The *stimulants are highly addictive* and are psychotoxic. Repeated administration may produce a state resembling an acute attack of schizophrenia.

Methylenedioxymethamphetamine (MDMA, 'ecstasy') is an amphetamine derivative with mixed stimulant and hallucinogenic properties, the latter action perhaps resulting from 5HT release. MDMA is widely abused as a 'recreational' drug, but it may produce psychiatric illness and occasionally severe acute hyperthermic reactions result in death.

Opioids

Diamorphine (heroin) and other opioids have a high misuse and dependence potential because of the intense sense of euphoria they produce when taken intravenously. Tolerance develops quickly in addicts and abrupt withdrawal of opioids results in a craving to take the drug, together with a withdrawal syndrome characterized by yawning, sweating, gooseflesh, tremor, irritability, anorexia, nausea and vomiting, which lasts 7–10 days. Withdrawal of longer-acting drugs, such as **methadone**, results in a more prolonged, but less intense, syndrome and the treatment of opioid withdrawal usually involves substitution with methadone followed by a slow 'tapering off'. **Clonidine** can suppress some components of the withdrawal syndrome, especially the nausea, vomiting and diarrhoea. **Lofexidine** (a clonidine analogue) is replacing clonidine as the standard non-substitute method for opioid detoxification because it is much less likely to cause hypotension and sedation. **Naltrexone**, an orally active opioid antagonist, prevents the euphoric action of opioids and is given to former addicts with the idea of preventing relapses.

The mechanisms underlying opioid dependence and tolerance are unknown. Chronic administration does not affect opioid receptors, but changes in second messengers may be important, e.g. in the *locus coeruleus*, μ-receptor activation inhibits adenylyl cyclase activity, but with chronic opioid administration the activity of the enzyme increases. Withdrawal of the inhibitory opioid then results in excessive cAMP production, which may contribute to the rebound (increase) of neuronal excitability.

Hallucinogens (*psychedelics*)

Lysergic acid diethylamide (LSD) and related drugs induce dramatic states of altered perception, vivid and unusual sensory experiences and feelings of ecstasy. Occasionally, LSD produces unwanted effects which include panic, frightening delusions and hallucinations. Usually the 'bad trip' fades away, but sometimes it returns later ('flashbacks').

Serotinergic systems may be important in the actions of LSD, which inhibits the firing of 5HT-containing neurones in the *raphe nuclei*, probably by stimulating $5HT_2$ inhibitory autoreceptors on these cells. Tolerance to LSD and related compounds occurs, and is associated with a downregulation of $5HT_2$ receptors. However, physical dependence to hallucinogens does not occur and there is no withdrawal syndrome.

Cannabis (*marijuana, hashish*). The main active constituent of cannabis is Δ'-tetrahydrocannabinol (THC). Cannabis has both hallucinogenic and depressant actions. It produces feelings of euphoria, relaxation and well-being. Cannabis is not dangerously addictive, but at least mild degrees of dependence may occur. Cannabis may cause acute psychotoxic effects that in some ways resemble an LSD 'bad trip'.

General depressants

Barbiturates have a high dependence potential and withdrawal can cause epileptic fits or a state resembling delirium tremens.

Alcohol has effects that resemble those of general anaesthetics. It inhibits presynaptic Ca^{2+} entry (and hence transmitter release) and potentiates GABA-mediated inhibition. Considerable tolerance occurs to alcohol, but the mechanisms involved are poorly understood. Presynaptic Ca^{2+} channels may increase in number, so that when alcohol is withdrawn transmitter release is abnormally high and this may contribute to the withdrawal syndrome.

Chronic heavy drinking leads to physical dependence and in the UK there are about 14 800 patients admitted each year to psychiatric hospitals for alcohol dependence and psychosis; brain damage and liver disease leading to cirrhosis are also common.

The physical withdrawal syndromes in humans range from a '*hangover*' to *epileptic fits* and the condition of '*delirium tremens*', in which the subject becomes agitated, confused and may have severe hallucinations. Alcohol (and barbiturate) withdrawal may require **chlormethiazole** or **benzodiazepine** administration to prevent convulsions. **Clonidine** may be helpful but does not protect against fits.

Tobacco (nicotine) is a highly addictive drug that is responsible for more damage to health in the UK than all other drugs (including alcohol) combined. Nicotine increases alertness, decreases irritability and decreases skeletal muscle tone (because Renshaw cells are stimulated). Tolerance occurs to some effects of nicotine, notably the nausea and vomiting seen in non-tolerant subjects. The *toxicity of tobacco* is due to the many chemicals in the smoke, some of which are known carcinogens. Serious diseases associated with chronic tobacco smoking include lung cancer, coronary heart disease and peripheral vascular disease. Smoking during pregnancy significantly reduces the birth weight of babies and increases perinatal mortality.

Withdrawal of tobacco may cause a syndrome (lasting 2–3 weeks) which includes 'craving' for tobacco, irritability, difficulty in concentration and often weight gain. These symptoms may be reduced by the use of **nicotine replacement products** (e.g. chewing gum, nasal sprays, skin patches). Unfortunately, the craving for tobacco leads to relapse in most people who try to give up smoking, even after myocardial infarction.

32 Non-steroidal anti-inflammatory drugs (NSAIDs)

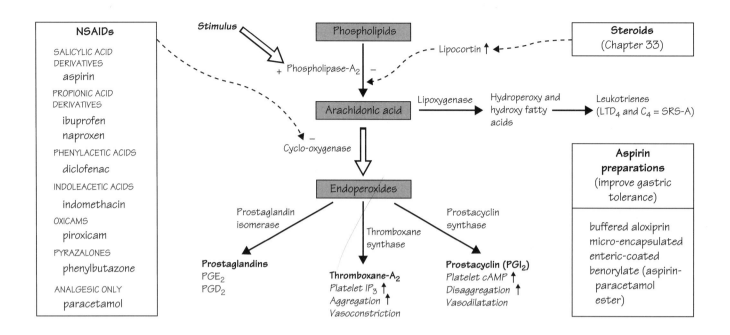

These drugs have *analgesic, antipyretic* and, at higher doses, *anti-inflammatory* actions. They are extensively used and in the UK almost a quarter of patients consulting their general practitioners have some form of 'rheumatic' complaint. These patients are frequently prescribed NSAIDs and additional millions of **aspirin**, **paracetamol** and **ibuprofen** tablets are bought over the counter for the self-treatment of headaches, dental pain, various musculoskeletal disorders, etc. They are not effective in the treatment of visceral pain (e.g. myocardial infarction, renal colic, acute abdomen), which requires opioid analgesics. However, NSAIDs are effective in certain types of severe pain (e.g. bone cancer). Aspirin has important antiplatelet activity (Chapter 19).

The NSAIDs form a chemically diverse group (left), but they all have the ability to **inhibit cyclo-oxygenase (COX)** (⟶) and the resulting inhibition of prostaglandin synthesis is largely responsible for their therapeutic effects. Unfortunately, the inhibition of prostaglandin synthesis in the gastric mucosa frequently results in *gastrointestinal damage* (dyspepsia, nausea and gastritis). More serious adverse effects include gastrointestinal bleeding and perforation. COX exists in the tissue as a constitutive isoform (COX-1) but at sites of inflammation cytokines stimulate the induction of a second isoform COX-2. Inhibition of COX-2 is probably responsible for the anti-inflammatory actions of NSAIDs, whilst inhibition of COX-1 may be responsible for their gastrointestinal toxicity. Currently used NSAIDs are somewhat selective for COX-1 but it is likely that selective COX-2 inhibitors may in the future provide less toxic NSAIDs.

Aspirin (acetylsalicylic acid) is the longest-standing NSAID and is an effective analgesic, with a duration of action of about 4 hours. Aspirin remains the drug of choice for many sorts of mild to moderate pain. Aspirin is well absorbed orally. As it is a weak acid ($pK_a = 3.5$), the acid pH of the stomach keeps a large fraction of aspirin non-ionized and therefore promotes absorption in the stomach, although much aspirin is absorbed via the large surface area of the upper small intestine. The absorbed aspirin is hydrolysed by esterases in the blood and tissues to salicylate (which is active) and acetic acid. Most salicylate is converted in the liver to water-soluble conjugates that are rapidly excreted by the kidney. Alkalinization of the urine ionizes the salicylate and, because this reduces its tubular reabsorption, excretion is increased.

Aspirin is a well-established drug in the treatment of inflammatory joint disease, but up to 50% of patients will not tolerate the adverse effects (nausea, vomiting, epigastric pain, tinnitis) caused by the high doses of soluble aspirin necessary to achieve an anti-inflammatory effect. Various preparations (bottom right) containing aspirin are designed to minimize its gastrointestinal effects, but for treating the symptoms of inflammatory joint disease (pain, stiffness and swelling) newer NSAIDs are generally preferred. NSAIDs seem to have similar effectiveness. However, there is considerable patient variation in response and so it is impossible to know which drug will be effective in an individual, although 60% of patients will respond to any drug. Since the propionic acid derivatives (e.g. **ibuprofen, naproxen**) are associated with fewer serious adverse effects, these are often tried first.

Paracetamol has no significant anti-inflammatory action, but is widely used as a mild analgesic when pain has no inflammatory component. It is well absorbed orally and does not cause gastric irritation. It has the disadvantage that, in overdosage, serious hepatotoxicity is likely to occur (Chapters 4 and 44).

Analgesic action. The analgesic action of NSAIDs is exerted both peripherally and centrally, but the peripheral actions predominate. Their analgesic action is usually associated with their anti-inflammatory action and results from the inhibition of prostaglandin synthesis in the inflamed tissues. Prostaglandins produce little pain by themselves, but potentiate the pain caused by other mediators of inflammation (e.g. histamine, bradykinin).

Anti-inflammatory action. The role of prostaglandins in inflammation is to produce vasodilatation and increased vascular permeability. However, inhibition of prostaglandin synthesis by NSAIDs attenuates rather than abolishes inflammation, because the drugs do not inhibit other mediators of inflammation. Nevertheless, the relatively modest anti-inflammatory actions of the NSAIDs give, to most patients with rheumatoid arthritis, some relief from pain, stiffness and swelling, but they do not alter the course of the disease.

Antipyretic action. NSAIDs do not reduce the normal body temperature or the elevated temperatures in heat stroke, which is due to hypothalamic malfunction. During fever, endogenous pyrogen (interleukin-1) is released from leucocytes and acts directly on the thermoregulatory centre in the hypothalamus to increase body temperature. This effect is associated with a rise in brain prostaglandins (which are pyrogenic). Aspirin prevents the temperature-raising effects of interleukin-1 by preventing the rise in brain prostaglandin levels.

Mechanism of action on COX. NSAIDs inhibit COX by several mechanisms. **Aspirin** acetylates a serine residue of the constitutive form of the enzyme, causing irreversible inhibition. This results from steric hindrance of access of substrate to the oxygenase active site. In contrast, other NSAIDs (including salicylate) are reversible competitive inhibitors of COX. **Paracetamol** acts at least partly by reducing cytoplasmic peroxide tone: peroxide is necessary to activate the haem enzyme to the ferryl form. In areas of acute inflammation, paracetamol is not very effective because neutrophils and monocytes produce high levels of H_2O_2 and lipid peroxide, which overcome the actions of the drug. However, paracetamol is an effective analgesic in conditions where leucocyte infiltration is absent or low.

Adverse effects of NSAIDs are common, partly because the drugs may be given in high doses for a long time and partly because they are widely used in elderly patients who are more susceptible to side effects.

Gastrointestinal tract. Damage to the mucosa of the gastrointestinal tract seems to be mainly a consequence of prostaglandin synthesis inhibition, rather than a directly erosive action of the drugs. Prostaglandins (PGE_2 and PGI_2) inhibit gastric acid secretion, increase blood flow though the gastric mucosa and have a cytoprotective action (PGE_2 and some analogues induce healing of peptic ulcer). By inhibiting prostaglandin formation, NSAIDs may cause ulceration by producing mucosal ischaemia and by impairing the protective mucus barrier, thus exposing the mucosa to the damaging effects of acid. **Misoprostol** is a PGE_1 derivative that is effective in preventing the gastrointestinal toxicity of NSAIDs. Its main indication is in patients with a history of peptic ulcer whose need for NSAID treatment is such that the analgesic cannot be withdrawn.

Nephrotoxicity. Prostaglandins PGE_2 and PGI_2 are powerful vasodilators synthesized in the renal medulla and glomeruli, respectively, and are involved in the control of renal blood flow and excretion of salt and water. Inhibition of renal prostaglandin synthesis may result in sodium retention, reduced renal blood flow and renal failure, especially in patients with conditions associated with vasoconstrictor catecholamine and angiotensin II release (e.g. congestive heart failure, cirrhosis). In addition, NSAIDs may cause interstitial nephritis and hyperkalaemia. Prolonged analgesic abuse over a period of years is associated with papillary necrosis and chronic renal failure.

Other adverse effects include bronchospasm, especially in asthmatics, skin rashes and other allergies.

OTHER NSAIDs

Propionic acids, such as **ibuprofen, fenbufen** and **naproxen,** are widely regarded as the drugs of first choice for the treatment of inflammatory joint disease, because they have the lowest incidence of side effects.

Indoleacetic acids. Indomethacin is one of the more effective agents, but has a higher incidence of adverse effects including ulceration, gastric bleeding, headaches and dizziness. It may also cause blood dyscrasias.

Oxicams. Piroxicam has a long half-life and only requires a single daily dose to be administered. It may be associated with a particularly high incidence of gastrointestinal bleeding in the elderly.

Pyrazolones. Phenylbutazone is an extremely potent anti-inflammatory agent, but has serious toxicity. It is restricted to hospital use for the treatment of intractable pain due to inflammatory arthritis such as ankylosing spondylitis because it sometimes causes fatal aplastic anaemia. **Azapropazone** does not cause bone marrow suppression but is the NSAID associated with the highest incidence of adverse effects. It is restricted for the treatment of patients where other drugs have failed.

GOUT

Gout is characterized by deposition of sodium urate crystals in the joint, causing painful arthritis. **Acute attacks** are treated with **indomethacin, naproxen, piroxicam** or other NSAIDs but *not with aspirin*, which raises plasma urate levels at low doses by inhibiting uric acid secretion in the renal tubules. **Colchicine** is effective in gout. It binds to tubulin in leucocytes and prevents their migration to the areas of uric acid deposition, and hence reduces the inflammatory responses. However, colchicine causes nausea, vomiting, diarrhoea and abdominal pain.

Prophylactic treatment of gout

Allopurinol lowers plasma urate by inhibiting xanthine oxidase, the enzyme responsible for urate synthesis. It is useful in patients with recurrent attacks of gout.

Uricosuric drugs, such as **sulphinpyrazone** and **probenecid,** inhibit renal tubular reabsorption of uric acid, increasing its excretion. Plenty of water should be taken to avoid the crystallization of urate in the urine. These drugs are less effective and more toxic than allopurinol. They are normally used in patients who cannot tolerate allopurinol.

33 Corticosteroids

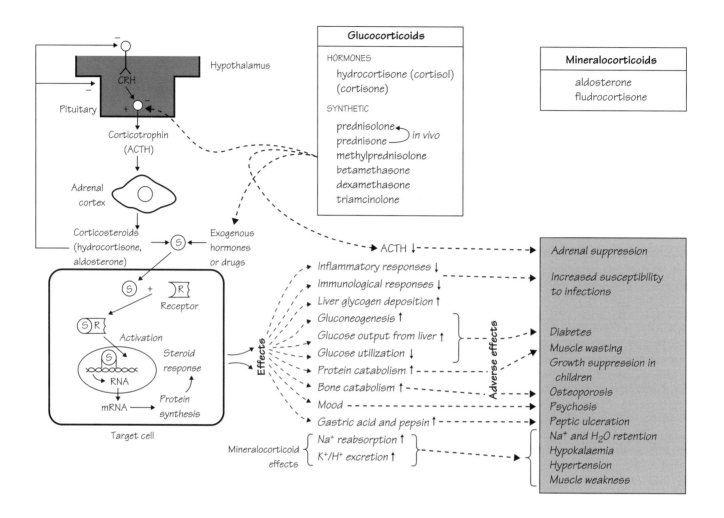

The adrenal cortex releases several steroid hormones into the circulation. They are divided by their actions into two classes. **Mineralocorticoids**, mainly aldosterone in humans, have salt-retaining activity and are synthesized in the cells of the zona glomerulosa. **Glucocorticoids**, mainly **cortisol** (hydrocortisone) in humans, affect carbohydrate and protein metabolism, but also have significant mineralocorticoid activity. They are synthesized in the cells of the zona fasciculata and zona reticularis.

The release of cortisol is controlled by a negative-feedback mechanism involving the hypothalamus and anterior pituitary (upper figure, ▨). Low plasma cortisol levels result in the release of corticotrophin (adrenocorticotrophic hormone, ACTH), which stimulates cortisol synthesis and release by activating adenylyl cyclase. Cyclic AMP then activates protein kinase A, which phosphorylates and increases the activity of cholesterylester hydrolase, the rate-limiting step in steroid synthesis. Aldosterone release is affected by ACTH but other factors (e.g. renin–angiotensin system, plasma potassium) are more important.

The steroids are examples of **gene-active** hormones. These produce their effects on cells (lower figure) by promoting the synthesis of specific messenger ribonucleic acid (mRNA) and so stimulate the synthesis of proteins which then produce the characteristic actions of the hormones (middle bottom).

The steroid **hormones** (**hydrocortisone** or **cortisone**) are given with a synthetic mineralocorticoid, usually **fludrocortisone** (top right), for replacement therapy in patients with adrenal insufficiency (e.g. in Addison's disease). For most therapeutic uses, **synthetic glucocorticoids** (top middle) have replaced the natural hormones, mainly because they have little or no salt-retaining activity.

Glucocorticoids (often **prednisolone**) are used to suppress inflammation, allergy and immune responses. Anti-inflammatory therapy is used in many diseases (e.g. rheumatoid arthritis, ulcerative colitis, bronchial asthma, severe inflammatory conditions of the eye and skin). Suppression of the immune system is of value in preventing rejection following tissue transplantation. Steroids are also used to suppress lymphopoiesis in patients with certain leukaemias and lymphomas.

Steroids can produce striking improvement in certain diseases, but high doses and prolonged use may cause **severe adverse effects** (right, ▨). These are usually predictable from the known actions of the drugs.

Corticotrophin releasing hormone (CRH) is a 41-amino-acid polypeptide whose action is enhanced by arginine vasopressin (ADH). It is produced in the hypothalamus and reaches the adenohypophysis in the hypothalamo–hypophysial portal system, where it stimulates the release of corticotrophin.

Corticotrophin (ACTH) is processed from a large-molecular-weight precursor, pro-opiomelanocortin (POMC), present in corticotroph cells of the adenohypophysis; its main action is to stimulate the synthesis and release of *cortisol* (hydrocortisone). POMC also contains the sequences for *β-lipotropin* (β-LPH) and *β-endorphin* which are concomitantly released into the blood. Corticotrophin is also believed to sensitize the zona glomerulosa to other stimuli, which cause aldosterone release (i.e. low plasma Na^+, high plasma K^+, angiotensin II).

GLUCOCORTICOIDS

Mechanisms of action. Cortisol (and synthetic glucocorticoids) diffuses into target cells and binds to a cytoplasmic glucocorticoid receptor that belongs to the superfamily of steroid, thyroid (Chapter 35) and retinoid receptors. The activated receptor–drug complex enters the nucleus and binds to a specific glucocorticoid regulatory element on target DNA molecules, initiating or inhibiting gene transcription. For most clinical purposes synthetic glucocorticoids are used because they have a *higher affinity for the receptor, are less rapidly inactivated, and have little or no salt-retaining properties.*

Hydrocortisone is used: (i) orally for replacement therapy; (ii) intravenously in shock and status asthmaticus; and (iii) topically (e.g. ointments in eczema, enemas in ulcerative colitis).

Prednisolone is the most widely used drug given orally in inflammatory and allergic diseases.

Betamethasone and dexamethasone are very potent and have no salt-retaining actions. This makes them especially useful for high-dose therapy in conditions, such as cerebral oedema, where water retention would be a disadvantage.

Beclomethasone, dipropionate and **budesonide** pass membranes poorly and are more active topically than when given orally. They are used in asthma (as an aerosol) and topically in severe eczema to provide a local anti-inflammatory action with minimal systemic effects.

Triamcinolone is used in severe asthma and by intra-articular injection for local inflammation of joints.

Effects. Glucocorticoids influence most cells in the body.

Metabolic effects. Glucocorticoids are essential for life, their most important action being to facilitate the conversion of protein to glycogen. Glucocorticoids inhibit protein synthesis and stimulate protein catabolism to amino acids. Gluconeogenesis, glycogen deposition and glucose release from the liver are stimulated but peripheral glucose uptake is inhibited. During fasting, glucocorticoids are vital to prevent (possibly fatal) hypoglycaemia.

Anti-inflammatory effects. Corticosteroids have profound anti-inflammatory effects and are widely used for this purpose. Inflammation is probably suppressed by several mechanisms. Circulating immunocompetent cells and macrophages are reduced and the formation of pro-inflammatory mediators, such as prostaglandins, leukotrienes and platelet activating factor (PAF), are inhibited. Steroids produce these latter effects by stimulating the synthesis in leucocytes of a protein ('lipocortin') that inhibits phospholipase A_2. This enzyme, located in the cell membrane, is activated in damaged cells and is responsible for the formation of arachidonic acid, the precursor of many inflammatory mediators (Chapter 32).

Immunosuppressive effects. Glucocorticoids depress monocyte/macrophage function and decrease circulating thymus-derived lymphocytes (T-cells), especially helper T_4 lymphocytes. The release of interleukins IL-1 and IL-2 (necessary to activate and stimulate lymphocyte proliferation) is inhibited. The transport of lymphocytes to the site of antigenic stimulation and the production of antibody is also inhibited.

Adverse effects

Glucocorticoids produce many adverse effects, especially with the high doses required for anti-inflammatory activity. (Similar effects are produced by the excess corticosteroids secreted in Cushing's syndrome.)

Metabolic effects. High doses quickly cause a rounded, plethoric face (moon face), and fat is redistributed from the extremities to the trunk and face. Purple striae and a tendency to bruise develop. Disturbed carbohydrate metabolism leads to hyperglycaemia and occasionally diabetes. Protein loss from skeletal muscles causes wasting and weakness. This cannot be remedied by dietary protein because protein synthesis is inhibited. An increase in bone catabolism may cause osteoporosis.

Fluid retention, hypokalaemia and hypertension may occur with compounds that have significant mineralocorticoid activity. Thus, hydrocortisone (and cortisone) are generally used only for replacement therapy in adrenal insufficiency.

Adrenal suppression. Steroid therapy suppresses corticotrophin secretion and this eventually leads to adrenal atrophy. It may take 6–12 months for normal adrenal function to recover once therapy is stopped. Since the patient's response to stress is suppressed, additional steroid must be administered in times of severe stress (e.g. surgery, infection). Steroid therapy must be withdrawn very gradually, because abrupt withdrawal causes adrenal insufficiency.

Infections. There is increased susceptibility to infections, which may progress unrecognized because the natural indicators of infection are inhibited.

Other complications include psychosis, cataracts, glaucoma, peptic ulceration and the reactivation of nascent infections (e.g. tuberculosis).

MINERALOCORTICOIDS

Fludrocortisone is given with hydrocortisone in adrenal insufficiency (e.g. Addison's disease or following adrenalectomy) because the latter drug does not possess sufficient salt-retaining activity.

34 Sex hormones and drugs

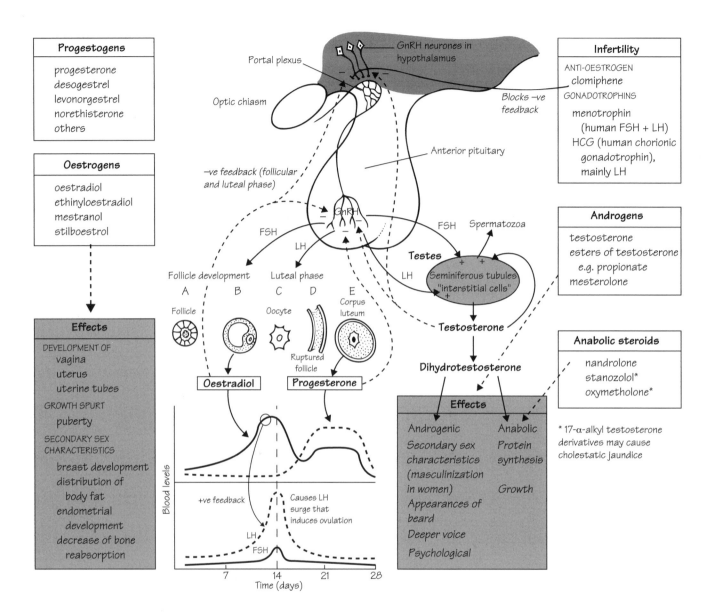

The ovaries and testes, in addition to producing gametes, also secrete hormones (mainly **oestrogens** and **androgens**, respectively). The secretion of oestrogens (mainly **oestradiol**) and androgens (mainly **testosterone**) requires **gonadotrophins** (luteinizing hormone (LH) and follicle stimulating hormone (FSH)), which are hormones released from the anterior pituitary (middle top). The release of LH and FSH is in turn controlled by the hypothalamus (top, ▨), which releases pulses of gonadotrophin-releasing hormone (GnRH).

In the **testes** (right, ⬭), spermatozoa are produced in the seminiferous tubules by a process requiring both FSH and *testosterone*, the latter hormone being synthesized in the interstitial cells in response to LH. Testosterone causes the changes that occur in the normal male at puberty (bottom right, shaded). **Androgens** (middle right) are used mainly for replacement therapy in castrated males or in males who are hypogonadal due to either pituitary or testicular disease. **Testosterone** is rapidly inactivated by the liver following oral administration, but synthetic androgens (e.g. **mesterolone**) are active orally. **Anabolic**

steroids (bottom right) have relatively little androgenic activity and are used to try and increase protein synthesis after major surgery and in chronic debilitating disease. The main adverse effects of androgens and, to a lesser extent, the anabolic steroids, is masculinization in women and prepubertal children and the suppression of FSH and LH.

In the **ovary**, FSH (and LH) stimulate follicular development (top left, A–B) and **oestradiol** synthesis by the granulosa cells of the follicle. In the early follicular phase, the low oestradiol level in the blood (middle left) exerts a negative feedback effect on FSH, ensuring that only the dominant follicle ripens. Midway through the cycle, oestradiol levels are high and this has a positive feedback effect on LH secretion, leading to the 'LH surge' (bottom left) that causes ovulation. These feedback effects of oestradiol are exerted on the hypothalamus (changing the amount of GnRH secreted) and the pituitary gland (altering its response to GnRH). The ruptured follicle (D) develops into the corpus luteum (E), which secretes oestrogen and progesterone (middle left) until the end of the cycle. During the follicular phase of the cycle, oestrogen stimulates endometrial proliferation. In the luteal phase, increased progesterone release stimulates the maturation and glandular development of the endometrium, which is then shed in the process of menstruation.

Oestrogens (middle left) have many effects (bottom left, shaded). They are used for replacement therapy in primary hypogonadism and in postmenopausal women to prevent hot flushes, atrophic vaginitis and osteoporosis. They are also used in a number of menstrual disorders (e.g. spasmodic dysmenorrhoea), and in combination with progestogens, as contraceptives. **Progestogens** (top left) are used mainly for hormonal contraception. Sex hormones and antagonists are used in the treatment of certain cancers (Chapter 43).

GnRH (**gonadorelin**) is a decapeptide that stimulates FSH and LH release from the anterior pituitary gland. Pulsatile infusions of GnRH are used to treat hypothalamic hypogonadism.

LH and **FSH** are glycoprotein hormones produced by the anterior pituitary. They regulate gonadal function.

INFERTILITY

In anovulatory women, infertility may be overcome, providing the ovary is capable of producing a mature ova and the appropriate steroids.

Clomiphene and **tamoxifen** are anti-oestrogens. They work by inhibiting the feedback inhibition of oestrogens in the hypothalamus and so increase FSH and LH release.

Gonadotrophins are used in women who lack appropriate pituitary function or do not respond to clomiphene therapy. Treatment starts with daily injections of **menotrophin** (LH and FSH in equal amounts) or **urofollitrophin** (FSH), followed by one or two large doses of **chorionic gonadotrophin** (mainly LH) to induce ovulation. Multiple births occur in 20–30% of pregnancies after treatment. In men, both gonadotrophins are given to stimulate spermatogenesis and androgen release.

TESTOSTERONE

The most important androgen in humans is testosterone. About 2% of testosterone in the plasma is free and in the skin, prostate, seminal vesicles and epididymis it is converted to dihydrotestosterone. Androgen deficiency is usually treated with depot injections of testosterone proprionate.

Effects. At puberty, androgens cause development of the secondary sexual characteristics in the male. In the adult male, large doses suppress the release of gonadotrophins and cause some atrophy of the interstitial tissue and tubules of the testes. In women, androgens cause changes, many of which are similar to those seen in the prepubertal male.

OESTROGENS

Oestradiol is the main oestrogen released by the human ovary. Synthetic oestrogens are more effective following oral administration.

Adverse effects (see oral contraceptives). The continuous administration of oestrogens for prolonged periods can cause abnormal endometrial hyperplasia, abnormal bleeding patterns, and is associated with an increased incidence of endometrial carcinoma. When a progestogen is given with the oestrogen, there is a decreased incidence of ovarian and endometrial cancers.

PROGESTOGENS

Progestogens are used for hormonal contraception and for producing long-term ovarian suppression for other purposes (e.g. dysmenorrhoea, endometriosis, hirsutism and bleeding disorders) when oestrogens are contraindicated.

ORAL CONTRACEPTIVES

Combination pills contain oestrogen and progestogen. They are taken for 20–21 days and discontinued for the following 6–7 days to allow menstruation to occur.

Mini-progestogen pills contain a low dose of progestogen and are taken continuously.

Only two oestrogens are used: **mestranol** and **ethinyloestradiol**. Enzyme-inducing drugs, e.g. phenobarbitone, carbamazepine, phenytoin and especially rifampicin, may cause failure of contraception.

Mechanism of action. Combination pills act by feedback inhibition on the hypothalamus to suppress GnRH and hence plasma gonadotrophin secretion, thereby blocking ovulation. These drugs also produce an endometrium that is unreceptive to implantation, alter Fallopian tube motility, and change the composition of cervical mucus. These latter effects are also produced by mini-progestogen pills and appear to be the basis of their contraceptive actions, since they only block ovulation in about 25% of women. Menstruation often ceases initially with mini-progestogens, but usually returns with prolonged administration. However, the length and duration of bleeding are very variable.

Adverse effects. *Non-life threatening* side effects that occur with both combination pills and mini-progestogens include breakthrough bleeding, weight gain, changes in libido, breast soreness, headache and nausea. Combination pills may also cause hirsutism, vaginal yeast infections and depression. About 20–30% of women will experience some of these effects and 10–15% will stop taking the pill because of them. The overall incidence of side effects is lower with mini-progestogens, but breakthrough bleeding and irregular menses are major complaints with these drugs.

Serious side effects are rare. They include cholestatic jaundice and a slightly greater incidence of thromboembolic disease, for which the oestrogen is apparently responsible. However, combined pills containing gestodene and desogestrol, are associated with a higher incidence of thromboembolism. A history of thromboembolism, cigarette smoking, hypertension and diabetes increases the thromboembolic risk of oral contraception.

'Abortion pill'. Progesterone supports endometrial nidation of the fertilized ovum and the progesterone antagonist, **mifepristone**, has been found to be highly effective in terminating early pregnancy when used with a prostaglandin cervical ripening agent (e.g. gemeprost pessaries). The main adverse effects are pain and bleeding.

35 Thyroid and antithyroid drugs

The thyroid gland secretes two iodinated hormones called **triiodothyronine (T_3)** and **thyroxine** (tetraiodothyronine, T_4), which are responsible for the optimal growth, development, function and maintenance of body tissues. Another hormone, **calcitonin**, is produced by the parafollicular cells and is involved in the regulation of calcium metabolism.

The synthesis of T_3 and T_4 requires **iodine**, which is normally ingested (as iodide) in the diet. An active, *thyrotrophin*-dependent pump (⇨) concentrates the **iodide** (I^-) in the follicular cells (centre figure) where, at the apical boundary, it is rapidly oxidized by peroxidase to the more reactive **iodine** (I^o). The iodine reacts with tyrosine residues present in thyroglobulin (Ⓣ) ('organification'), and units of T_3 (◇) and T_4 (◆) are formed. The thyroglobulin containing these iodothyronines is stored in the follicles as colloid (□).

The release of T_3 and T_4 is controlled by a negative feedback system (top figure). When the circulating levels of T_3 and T_4 fall, **thyrotrophin (TSH)** is released from the anterior pituitary gland and stimulates the transport of colloid (by endocytosis) into the follicular cells. Then, the colloid droplets fuse with lysosomes, and protease enzymes degrade the thyroglobulin, releasing T_3 (◇) and T_4 (◆) into the circulation. Both thyroid hormones act on **receptors (R)** in the plasma membrane and on intracellular receptors (bottom figure) to produce a variety of actions (right).

Thyroid hyperfunction and hypofunction occur in about 2% of the population and, together with diabetes mellitus (2–3% of the population), are the most common endocrine disorders. In **Graves' disease**, hyperthyroidism is produced by an antibody that causes prolonged activation of the TSH receptors and results in excessive secretion of T_3 and T_4. Thyroid activity can be reduced with drugs that reduce hormone synthesis (left), or by the destruction of the gland with radiation (using ^{131}I) or surgery. Hyperthyroidism often causes increased sympathetic effects, which can be blocked with β-adrenoceptor antagonists (e.g. propranolol). Graves' disease is often associated with ophthalmopathy, which is often difficult to control and may be a distinct organ-specific autoimmune disease.

Primary hypothyroidism (**myxoedema**) probably results in most cases from a cell-mediated immune response directed against the thyroid follicular cells. Thyroxine is the drug of choice for replacement therapy (top right).

Thyrotrophin-releasing hormone (TRH) is a tripeptide synthesized in the hypothalamus and transported in the capillaries of the pituitary portal venous system to the pituitary gland, where it stimulates TSH synthesis and release.

TSH. Thyrotrophin is a glycoprotein hormone that is released from the pituitary gland (adenohypophysis) and by activation of adenylyl cyclase stimulates the synthesis and release of hormones from the thyroid gland. In hypothyroidism or (rarely) iodine deficiency, abnormally high levels of TSH result in the enlargement of the thyroid gland (goitre).

T_3 and T_4. Triiodothyronine and thyroxine (tetraiodothyronine) enter the circulation, where they are transported largely bound to plasma proteins (99.5% and 99.95%, respectively). The thyroid only contributes about 20% of the unbound circulating T_3, the remainder being produced by the *peripheral conversion* of T_4 to T_3. T_4 may also be deiodinated to inactive reverse T_3 according to the demands of the tissues. T_4 seems to be mainly a prohormone of T_3.

Actions. The mechanisms of action of the thyroid hormones are not fully understood, but are thought to involve high-affinity binding sites (receptors) in the *plasma membrane, mitochondria* and *nucleus*. These receptor–hormone interactions result in a variety of effects, including increased protein synthesis and an increase in energy metabolism. Most **receptors** are intracellular. The nuclear receptors for T_3 (and steroids and vitamin D) are coded for by a superfamily of genes related to the *cis*-oncogenes. Free T_3/T_4 enters the cell by a carrier mechanism and most T_4 is converted to T_3 (or rT_3), which binds to the C-terminus of the receptor and induces a conformation change in its DNA binding site. This permits the activated receptor to interact with a thyroid hormone regulatory element in the target DNA molecules. Hence, gene transcription and protein synthesis are stimulated or repressed.

HYPERTHYROIDISM (THYROTOXICOSIS)

The basal metabolic rate is increased, causing heat intolerance, arrhythmias and increased appetite. The skin is warm and moist. There is increased nervousness and hyperkinesia. Sympathetic overactivity causes tachycardia, sweating and tremor. Angina and high-output heart failure may occur. The upper eyelids are retracted, causing a wide stare.

Traditionally, young patients have been treated with antithyroid drugs and, if the condition relapses, subtotal thyroidectomy. Patients over about 40 years of age have been given radioiodine therapy. Nowadays, young patients may be given ^{131}I and carbimazole may be given long term.

ANTITHYROID DRUGS

Thionamides possess a thiocarbamide group (S=C–N) that is essential for their activity. They prevent the synthesis of thyroid hormones by competitively inhibiting the peroxidase-catalysed reactions necessary for iodine organification. They also block the coupling of the iodotyrosine, especially diiodothyronine formation. Thionamides may be immunosuppressive, but this is controversial. All the antithyroid drugs are administered orally and are accumulated in the thyroid gland. Their onset of action is delayed until the preformed hormones are depleted, a process that may take 3–4 weeks.

Carbimazole is rapidly converted to methimazole *in vivo*. The aim is to render the patient euthyroid and then to give a reduced dose for maintenance. It is often possible to cease treatment after 1 or 2 years. Side effects include rashes and, rarely, agranulocytosis (warn patients to report a sore throat).

Propylthiouracil is usually reserved for patients intolerant to carbimazole. It is associated with a higher incidence of agranulocytosis (0.4%) than carbimazole (0.1%). In addition to inhibiting hormone synthesis, propylthiouracil also inhibits the peripheral deiodination of T_4 and perhaps has an immunosuppressive action.

Iodine. Iodides have several poorly understood actions on the thyroid. They inhibit organification and hormone release. In addition, iodide decreases the size and vascularity of the hyperplastic gland, effects which are useful in the preparation of patients for thyroidectomy. In 'pharmacological' doses, the main effect of iodides is to inhibit hormone release (possibly by inhibition of thyroglobulin proteolysis) and, because thyrotoxic symptoms are reduced relatively quickly (2–7 days), iodine is valuable in the treatment of thyroid storm (thyrotoxic crisis). Iodine cannot be used for the long-term treatment of hyperthyroidism because its antithyroid action tends to diminish.

Propranolol or atenolol can reduce the heart rate and other sympathetic manifestations of hyperthyroidism and provide partial relief of symptoms until full control is achieved with carbimazole. It is useful in the preoperative preparation of patients undergoing thyroidectomy. Propranolol is also used together with hydrocortisone, iodine and carbimazole in thyrotoxic crisis (thyroid storm).

HYPOTHYROIDISM

Tiredness and lethargy are the most common symptoms. Other effects include depression of the basal metabolic rate, appetite and cardiac output. Low-output heart failure may occur. The skin is dry. Thyroid hormone deprivation in early life results in irreversible mental retardation and dwarfism (cretinism), and to prevent this all newborn infants are screened and replacement therapy given from birth.

REPLACEMENT THERAPY

Thyroxine administered orally is the treatment of choice. Synthetic T_4 is the sodium salt of L-thyroxine. Its effects are delayed until the plasma protein and tissue binding sites are occupied. Treatment can be assessed by monitoring plasma TSH levels, which fall to normal when the optimum dose is achieved.

Liothyronine is the sodium salt of T_3 and because it is less protein bound, it acts more quickly than T_4. The main use of T_3 is in hypothyroid coma, when it is given (together with hydrocortisone) by intravenous injection.

36 Antidiabetic agents

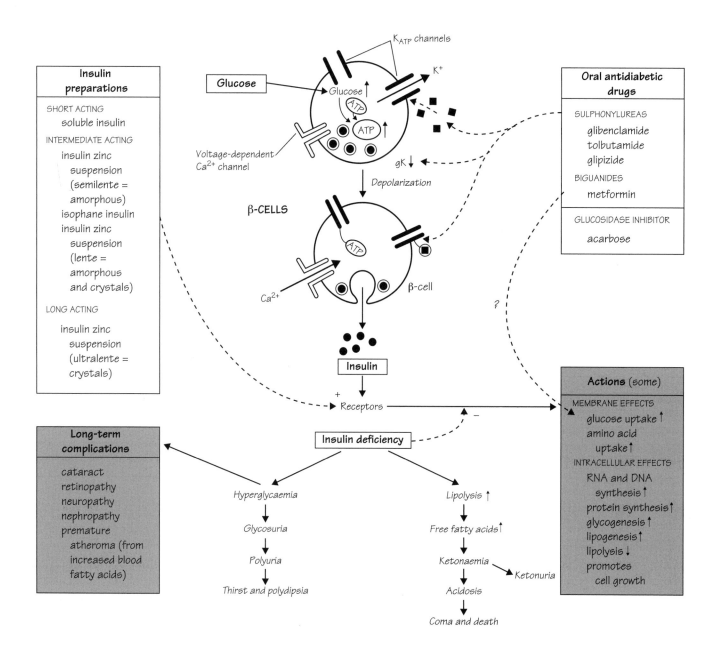

Insulin is a hormone secreted by the β-cells of the islets of Langerhans in the pancreas (top). Various stimuli **release** insulin (●) from storage granules (◉) in the β-cells, but the most potent stimulus is a rise in plasma glucose (hyperglycaemia). Insulin binds to specific **receptors** in the cell membranes, initiating a number of actions (bottom right, shaded) including an increase of glucose uptake by muscle, liver and adipose tissue.

In **diabetes mellitus** there is a relative or total absence of insulin, which causes reduced glucose uptake by insulin-sensitive tissues and has serious consequences (middle bottom). Lipolysis and muscle proteolysis result in weight loss and weakness. The blood levels of free fatty acids and glycerol rise. An excess of acetyl-CoA is produced in the liver and converted to *acetoacetic acid*, which is then either reduced to *β-hydroxybutyric* acid or decarboxylated to *acetone*. These 'ketone

bodies' accumulate in the blood, causing an acidosis (ketoacidosis). About 25% of diabetics have a severe deficiency of insulin. This **type I** or **insulin-dependent diabetes** is associated with HLA antigens and immunological selective β-cell destruction. In these patients, *ketosis* is common and insulin is required. Various **insulin preparations** (top left) and **regimens** are used. There is evidence that metabolic control early in the course of the disease may prevent or delay the onset of diabetic complications (bottom left, shaded). In **type II** or **non-insulin-dependent diabetes** the aetiology is unknown, but a strong genetic component is present. There is a resistance to circulating insulin, which does, however, protect the patient from ketosis. There is a reduction in the number of insulin receptors and this is often associated with obesity. Loss of weight (diet and exercise) reduces insulin 'resistance' and controls about one-third of type II diabetics. Another one-third of type

II diabetics are controlled by diet together with **oral antidiabetic drugs** (top right). The **sulphonylureas** (■) close K_{ATP} channels (middle), causing depolarization of the β-cells and increased insulin release. **Acarbose** is a new type of drug that delays the absorption of glucose following a meal. Type II diabetics not controlled by diet and oral antidiabetic drugs require insulin injections. These tend to be the thinner patients who lack the first phase insulin response.

INSULIN

Insulin is a polypeptide containing 51 amino acids arranged in two chains (A and B) linked by disulphide bridges. A precursor, called pro-insulin, is hydrolysed inside storage granules to form insulin and a residual C-peptide. The granules store insulin as crystals containing zinc and insulin.

Release. Glucose is the most potent stimulus for insulin release from islet β-cells. There is a continuous basal secretion with surges at feeding times. The β-cells possess K^+ channels that are regulated by intracellular ATP (K_{ATP} channels). When the blood glucose increases, more glucose enters the β-cells and its metabolism results in an increase in intracellular ATP, which closes the K_{ATP} channels. The resulting depolarization of the β-cell initiates an influx of Ca^{2+} ions through voltage-sensitive Ca^{2+} channels and this triggers insulin release.

Insulin receptors are membrane-spanning glycoproteins consisting of two α-subunits and two β-subunits linked covalently by disulphide bonds. After insulin binds to the α-subunit, the insulin–receptor complex enters the cell, where it is eventually destroyed by lysosomal enzymes. The internalization of the insulin–receptor complex may underlie the *downregulation* of receptors that is produced by high levels of insulin (e.g. in obese subjects). The mechanisms linking insulin–receptor activation to the actions of insulin are not understood, but a tyrosine kinase activity of the β-subunit and its autophosphorylation seem essential for insulin action.

INSULIN PREPARATIONS

Most diabetics in the UK are now treated with human insulin prepared by recombinant DNA technology, although some patients remain on insulin prepared from porcine or beef pancreas. Insulin is administered by subcutaneous injection and its rate of *absorption* can be prolonged by *increasing the particle size* (i.e. crystals slower than amorphous) or by *complexing the insulin with zinc or protamine*. Insulin preparations are classified traditionally into *short*, *intermediate* and *long acting*.

Short-acting insulin. Soluble insulin is a simple solution of insulin. (Onset 30 minutes, peak activity 2–4 hours, duration up to 8 hours). It can be administered intravenously in hyperglycaemic emergencies but its effects only last for 30 minutes by this route.

Intermediate and long-acting insulins. *Insulins* have a duration of action between 16 and 35 hours. **Semilente** is a suspension of amorphous insulin zinc. **Lente** is a mixture of amorphous insulin zinc (30%) and insulin zinc crystals (70%), the latter prolonging the duration of this preparation.

Isophane insulin (NPH) is a complex of protamine and insulin. The mixture is such that no free binding sites remain on the protamine. After injection, proteolytic enzymes degrade the protamine and the insulin is absorbed. The duration of NPH is similar to that of *lente* (about 20 hours).

Biphasic fixed mixtures contain various proportions of soluble and isophane insulin (e.g. 30% soluble and 70% isophane). The soluble component gives a rapid onset and the isophane insulin prolongs the action.

Ultralente is a suspension of poorly soluble insulin zinc crystals that has a duration up to 35 hours. The long duration of *ultralente* can lead to insulin accumulation and dangerous hypoglycaemia.

Adverse effects

Hypoglycaemia due to insulin overdose or inadequate calorific intake is the most common and most serious complication of insulin treatment. When severe, coma and death will occur if the patient is not treated with glucose (intravenously if unconscious). *Insulin antibodies.* All insulins are immunogenic to some extent (bovine most) but immunological resistance to insulin is rare. *Lipohypertrophy* is common with all preparations of insulin but local allergic reactions at the injection site are now very rare.

Insulin regimens. Most type I diabetic patients use a regimen involving a short-acting insulin mixed with intermediate-acting insulin injected subcutaneously twice daily, before breakfast and before the evening meal. More demanding, intensive control regimens, designed to produce near-normoglycaemia, reduce diabetic complications (one such regimen is an injection of intermediate-acting insulin, to provide a background level of insulin, and soluble insulin three times a day before meals).

ORAL ANTIDIABETIC DRUGS

Sulphonylureas are indicated in patients (especially those near their ideal weight) in whom diet fails to control the hyperglycaemia, but in about 30% control is not achieved with these drugs. These agents stimulate insulin release from the pancreatic islets and so the patient must have *partially functional β-cells* for these drugs to be of use. **Glibenclamide** is widely used and is sometimes effective when tolbutamide fails. If glibenclamide fails, other drugs are unlikely to be effective. **Tolbutamide** is less potent than glibenclamide but its short duration of action makes it the preferred drug in the elderly.

Adverse effects. Gastrointestinal disturbances and rashes occur, but are rare. Hypoglycaemia and hypoglycaemic coma may be induced by longer-acting drugs, *especially in elderly patients*. Sulphonylureas are contraindicated in severe (especially ketotic) hyperglycaemia, surgery and major illness, when insulin should be given.

Biguanides. Metformin acts peripherally to increase glucose uptake by an unknown mechanism. As it does not increase insulin release, it rarely causes hypoglycaemia. Adverse effects include nausea, vomiting, diarrhoea and, very occasionally, fatal lactic acidosis.

Acarbose inhibits intestinal α-glycosidases, delaying the digestion of starch and sucrose. It is taken with meals and lowers the postprandial increase of blood glucose. Its main side effect is flatulence.

79

37 Antimicrobial drugs that inhibit nucleic acid synthesis: sulphonamides, trimethoprim, quinolones and nitroimidazoles

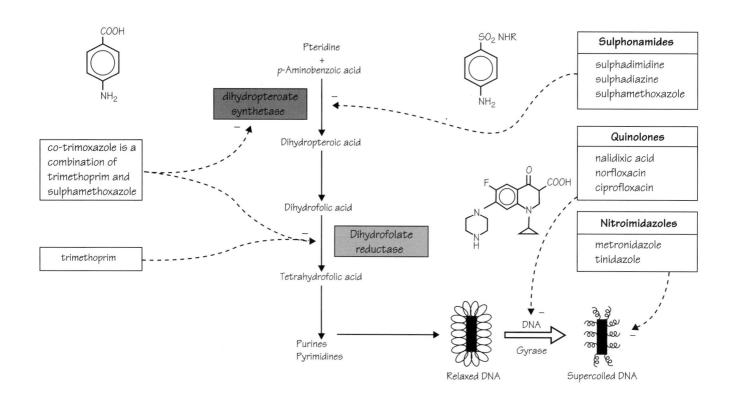

The sulphonamides were the first drugs found to be effective in the treatment of systemic infections. However, they are now of little importance because of the development of more effective agents that are less toxic. Also, many organisms have developed **resistance** to sulphonamides. Their principal use alone is in the treatment of urinary tract infections caused by sensitive Gram-positive or Gram-negative organisms.*

There are many sulphonamides and a few examples are given together with their general structure (top right). They are structural analogues of *p*-aminobenzoic acid (top left), which is essential for folic acid synthesis in bacteria. The **selective toxicity** of the sulphonamides depends on the fact that mammalian cells take up folate supplied in the diet, but susceptible bacteria lack this ability and must synthesize folate. Sulphonamides competitively inhibit the enzyme dihydropteroate synthetase (■), and prevent the production of folate required for the synthesis of DNA. The sulphonamides are **bacteriostatic** agents. Their most important side effects are rashes (common), renal failure and various blood dyscrasias.

Trimethoprim (bottom left) acts on the same metabolic pathway as sulphonamides, but is an inhibitor of dihydrofolate reductase (▨). It is selectively toxic because its affinity for the bacterial enzyme is

50 000 times greater than its affinity for the human enzyme. Trimethoprim is widely used in urinary tract infections. A combination of trimethoprim and sulphamethoxazole (**co-trimoxazole**) (left) may produce a synergistic action and increased activity against certain bacteria. Co-trimoxazole is used mainly in the treatment of respiratory infections.

The **4-quinolones** (middle right) inhibit DNA gyrase, an enzyme that compresses bacterial DNA into supercoils (⇨). Inhibition of DNA gyrase is believed to lead to unwinding of the supercoils and, ultimately, cell death. Eukaryotic cells do not contain DNA gyrase. **Ciprofloxacin** is a broad-spectrum antibacterial agent. Important properties of the quinolones are their good penetration into tissues and cells (cf. penicillins), their effectiveness when given orally, and their relatively low toxicity.

The **5-nitroimidazoles**, e.g. **metronidazole** (bottom right) have a very wide spectrum and are active against anaerobic bacteria and some protozoa (Chapter 42). The drug diffuses into the organism where the nitro-group is reduced. During this reduction process, chemically reactive intermediates are formed that inhibit DNA synthesis and/or damage DNA, impairing its function.

---

*Bacteria are classified by their shape (cocci are spherical, bacilli are rod-shaped) and many by whether (Gram-positive) or not (Gram-negative) they remain stained with methyl violet after washing with acetone. The retention or not of methyl violet reflects important differences in the bacterial cell walls.

Selective toxicity. The use of chemicals to try and eradicate parasites, bacteria, viruses or cancer cells in the body is called chemotherapy. It depends on the drugs being selectively toxic, i.e. toxic to the cells of the parasite, but not (too) toxic to the human host. Bacteria have many biochemical differences from human cells, and some antibacterial drugs are strikingly non-toxic to humans. On the other hand, because cancer cells are so similar to normal cells, most anticancer drugs show little selective toxicity and therefore produce serious adverse effects (Chapter 43).

Bacteriostatic agents inhibit bacterial growth, whilst **bactericidal agents** actually kill the organism. This distinction is not usually important clinically, as host–defence mechanisms are involved in the final elimination of bacterial pathogens. An exception is the treatment of infections in immunocompromised patients (acquired immune deficiency syndrome (AIDS), corticosteroids, anticancer and immunosuppressant drugs), when a bactericidal agent should be used.

Resistance to antimicrobial drugs can be acquired or innate. In the latter case, an entire bacterial species may be resistant to a drug before its introduction. For example, *Pseudomonas aeruginosa* has always been resistant to flucloxacillin. More serious clinically is **acquired resistance**, where bacteria that were once sensitive to a drug become resistant. Mechanisms responsible for resistance to antimicrobial drugs include the following.
1   Inactivating enzymes that destroy the drug, e.g. β-lactamases produced by many staphylococci inactivate most penicillins and many cephalosporins.
2   Decreased drug accumulation. Tetracycline resistance occurs where the bacterial cell membrane becomes impermeable to the drug or there is increased efflux.
3   Alteration of binding sites. Aminoglycosides and erythromycin bind to bacterial ribosomes and inhibit protein synthesis. In resistant organisms, the sites of drug binding may be modified so that they no longer have affinity for the drugs.
4   Development of alternative metabolic pathways. Bacteria can become resistant to sulphonamides and trimethoprim because they produce modified dihydropteroate synthetase and dihydrofolate reductase enzymes, respectively, which have little or no affinity for the drugs.
   Antibiotic-resistant bacterial populations can develop in several ways.
1   Selection. Within a population there will be some bacteria with acquired resistance. The drug then eliminates the sensitive organisms and the resistant forms proliferate.
2   Transferred resistance. Here, the gene that codes for the resistance mechanism is transferred from one organism to another. The antibiotic resistance genes may be carried in **plasmids**, which are small autonomously replicating extrachromosomal pieces of DNA within the bacteria. The plasmids (and therefore antibiotic resistance) can be transferred from one organism to another by *conjugation* (the formation of a tube between the organisms). Many Gram-negative and some Gram-positive bacteria can conjugate. In *transduction*, plasmid DNA is enclosed in a bacterial virus (bacteriophage) and transferred to another organism of the same species. This is a relatively ineffective method of transfer, but is clinically important in the transfer of resistance genes between strains of staphylococci and streptococci.

SULPHONAMIDES

Sulphadimidine and **sulphadiazine** are well absorbed following oral administration. These drugs were used to treat 'simple' urinary tract infections but many *Escherichia coli*† strains are resistant and much less toxic drugs are now available.

Adverse effects. The most common side effects are allergic reactions and include skin rashes (morbilliform or urticarial), sometimes with a fever. Much less common are more serious reactions, e.g. the Stevens–Johnson syndrome, which is a form of erythema multiforme with a high mortality rate. Sulphonamides with a low solubility, such as sulphadiazine, may crystallize from the urine in the kidneys (crystalluria), causing damage. This can be prevented by making the urine alkaline with sodium bicarbonate and maintaining a high fluid intake. It is not a problem with more soluble sulphonamides, such as sulphamethoxazole. Various blood dyscrasias may occur, rarely, including agranulocytosis, aplastic anaemia and haemolytic anaemia (especially in patients with glucose-6-phosphodehydrogenase deficiency).

Trimethoprim is well absorbed orally and is effective in most patients with simple lower urinary tract infections. It is sometimes used for respiratory tract infections, but it has relatively poor activity against *Streptococcus pneumoniae* and *Streptococcus pyogenes*. **Co-trimoxazole (trimethoprim** combined with **sulphamethoxazole**). Because the side effects of co-trimoxazole are mainly the same as those of the sulphonamide, its use is now largely restricted to treating patients with *Pneumocystis carinii* pneumonia, *nocardiasis* and toxoplasmosis.

QUINOLONES

Nalidixic acid was the first 4-quinolone found to have antibacterial activity, but it does not achieve systemic antibacterial levels and has been used only for urinary tract infections. **Ciprofloxacin** has a 6-fluoro substituent that confers greatly enhanced antibacterial potency against both Gram-positive and especially Gram-negative organisms, including *E. coli*, *Pseudomonas aeruginosa*, salmonella and campylobacter. So far, resistance is uncommon. Ciprofloxacin is well absorbed orally and can be given intravenously. It is eliminated, largely unchanged, mainly by the kidneys. Side effects are infrequent but include nausea, vomiting, rashes, dizziness and headache. Convulsions may occur because the quinolones are GABA antagonists. **Norfloxacin** has no systemic activity. It is concentrated in the urine and is a second-line drug in urinary tract infections.

5-NITROIMIDAZOLES

Metronidazole is well absorbed orally and can be given intravenously. It is active against most anaerobic bacteria including *Bacteroides* species. Metronidazole is the drug of choice in certain protozoal infections, i.e. *Entamoeba histolytica*, *Giardia lamblia*, *Trichomonas vaginalis* (Chapter 42). Side effects include gastrointestinal disturbances. **Tinidazole** has similar actions to metronidazole but has a longer duration of action.

---

† *E. coli* is a Gram-negative rod and is the most common cause of urinary tract infections.

38 Antimicrobial drugs that inhibit cell wall synthesis: penicillins, cephalosporins and vancomycin

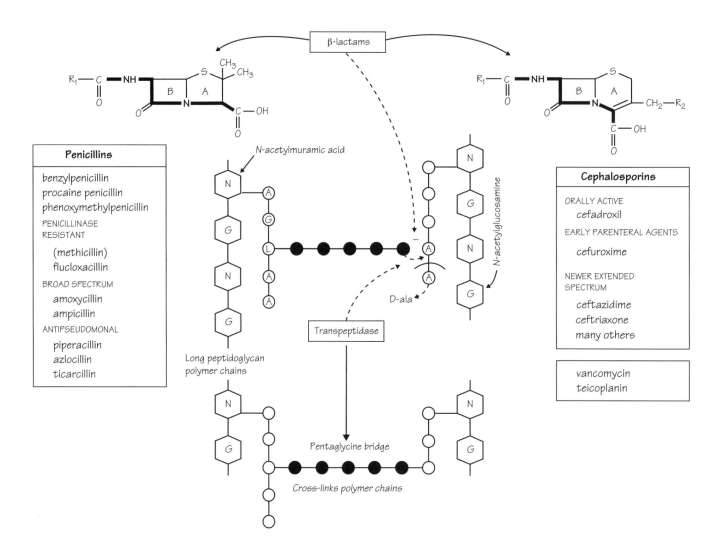

The structures of the penicillins (top left) and cephalosporins (top right) share the common feature of a β-lactam ring (B), the integrity of which is essential for antimicrobial activity. Modification of groups R_1 and R_2 have resulted in many semisynthetic antibiotics, some of which are acid resistant (and orally active), have a wide spectrum of antimicrobial activity, or are resistant to bacterial β-lactamases. The penicillins (left) are the most important antibiotics;* the cephalosporins (right) have few specific indications. The β-lactam antibiotics are **bactericidal**. They produce their antimicrobial action by preventing the cross-linkage between the linear peptidoglycan polymer chains that make up the cell wall, e.g. by a pentaglycine bridge (●). This action is because a part of their structure (▬) resembles the D-alanyl-D-alanine of the peptide chains of the bacterial cell wall.

Benzylpenicillin was the first of the penicillins and remains important, but it is largely destroyed by gastric acid and must be given by injection. **Phenoxymethylpenicillin** has a similar antimicrobial spec-

trum, but is active orally. Many bacteria (including most staphylococci) are resistant to benzylpenicillin because they produce enzymes (β-lactamases, penicillinase) that open the β-lactam ring. The genetic control of β-lactamases often resides in transmissible plasmids (Chapter 37). Some penicillins, e.g. **flucloxacillin**, are effective against β-lactamase-producing staphylococci. Gram-negative, but not Gram-positive, bacteria possess an outer phospholipid membrane that may confer penicillin resistance by hindering access of the drugs to the cell wall. The **broad-spectrum** penicillins, such as **amoxycillin** and **ampicillin**, are more hydrophilic than benzylpenicillin and are active against some Gram-negative bacteria because they can pass through pores in the outer phospholipid membrane. Penicillinase-producing organisms are resistant to amoxycillin and ampicillin. The **antipseudomonal penicillins** (bottom left) are used mainly for the treatment of serious infections caused by *Pseudomonas aeruginosa*.†

---

*Antibiotics are chemotherapeutic agents made by living micro-organisms rather than by chemical synthesis.

†*Pseudomonas aeruginosa* is a Gram-negative bacillus resistant to many antibiotics. It can cause serious opportunistic infections including pneumonia and septicaemia.

Penicillins have a very low toxicity, but high concentrations (renal failure, intrathecal administration) may produce encephalopathy, which can be fatal. **Hypersensitivity** is the most important side effect of the penicillins, which may cause rashes and, rarely, **anaphylactic reactions** that are fatal in about 10% of cases.

PENICILLINS

Benzylpenicillin remains one of the most useful antibiotics but it has a 'narrow spectrum' of activity, mainly against Gram-positive organisms. Benzylpenicillin is effective for treating pneumococcal, streptococcal, meningococcal and leptospiral infections. It is also valuable for the prophylaxis of clostridial gas gangrene. Most *Staphylococcus aureus*‡ now produces penicillinase. Benzylpenicillin is acid labile and is therefore poorly absorbed orally. It is given by intramuscular injection, but large doses are painful and are given intravenously. Penicillin diffuses widely though the body tissues, but penetration into the brain is poor, except when the meninges are inflamed. Following intramuscular injection, peak plasma levels occur after 15–30 minutes and the drug is rapidly excreted (largely unchanged) by the kidneys. The elimination half-life ($t_{1/2}$) is normally 30 minutes, but is prolonged to about 10 hours in anuria. The renal tubular secretion of penicillin can be inhibited by organic acids such as **probenecid** and this results in higher and more prolonged plasma concentrations.

Procaine penicillin is a sparingly soluble salt of benzylpenicillin; it is given by intramuscular injection and has a prolonged action. It is given in combination with benzylpenicillin (**bicillin**) for the treatment of syphilis.

Phenoxymethylpenicillin has the same spectrum as benzylpenicillin, but is less active. It is acid stable and is given orally. However, its absorption is variable and it is only useful for very sensitive organisms, where a rapid action is unnecessary (streptococcal tonsillitis). Phenoxymethylpenicillin is useful in the prophylaxis of rheumatic fever.

Penicillinase-resistant penicillins—flucloxacillin. Flucloxacillin is indicated in infections due to penicillinase-producing penicillin-resistant staphylococci. It is a semisynthetic penicillin and is resistant to penicillinase because an isoxazolyl group at R_1 sterically hinders access of the enzyme to the β-lactam ring. Flucloxacillin is less effective than benzylpenicillin and should only be used in infections due to penicillinase-producing staphylococci (which includes about 90% of hospital-acquired staphylococcal infections). Flucloxacillin is well absorbed orally, but in severe infections it should be given by injection and not be used alone. Epidemic strains of *Staphylococcus aureus* resistant to methicillin (MRSA), flucloxacillin and other antibiotics are an increasing problem, especially in hospitals. Such infections are best treated with intravenous vancomycin.

Broad-spectrum penicillins. Ampicillin and **amoxycillin** are active against non-β-lactamase-producing Gram-positive bacteria, and because they diffuse into Gram-negative bacteria more readily than benzylpenicillin, they are also active against many strains of *Escherichia coli*, *Haemophilus influenzae* and *Salmonella*. For oral administration, amoxycillin is the drug of choice, because it is better absorbed than ampicillin, which should be given parentally. Amoxycillin and ampicillin are inactivated by penicillinase-producing bacteria. Organisms that are resistant to amoxycillin include most *Staphylococcus aureus*, 50% of *Escherichia coli* strains and up to 15% of *Haemophilus influenzae* strains. Many bacterial β-lactamases are inhibited by **clavulanic acid**, and a mixture of this inhibitor with **amoxycillin** (**co-amoxiclav**) results in the antibiotic being effective against penicillinase-producing organisms. Co-amoxiclav is indicated in respiratory and urinary tract infections, which are confirmed resistant to amoxycillin.

Antipseudomonal penicillins. Piperacillin, **azlocillin** and **ticarcillin** are given by injection for serious infections with Gram-negative bacteria, especially *Pseudomonas aeruginosa*. They can be combined with aminoglycosides for the initial treatment of serious infection (e.g. septicaemia, endocarditis) when the bacterial cause has not been identified.

CEPHALOSPORINS

The cephalosporin antibiotics are used for the treatment of meningitis, pneumonia and septicaemia. The cephalosporins have the same mechanism of action as, and similar pharmacology to, penicillin. They may produce allergic reactions and cross-sensitivity to penicillin may occur. They are excreted mainly by the kidneys and their actions can be prolonged with probenecid. They all have a similar broad spectrum of antibacterial activity, although individual drugs have different activity against certain bacteria. **Cefadroxil** is administered orally and is used in urinary tract infections where the organisms are resistant to other antibiotics. **Cefuroxime** is given by injection often as a prophylactic in surgery (usually with metronidazole to provide cover against anaerobes). Cefuroxime is resistant to inactivation by bacterial β-lactamases and is used in serious infections when other antibiotics are ineffective. **Ceftazidime** has an increased range of activity against Gram-negative bacteria including *Pseudomonas aeruginosa*, but is less active than cefuroxime against Gram-positive organisms (e.g. *Staphylococcus aureus*). It reaches the central nervous system and is used in meningitis due to Gram-negative organisms. **Ceftriaxone** has a longer half-life than other cephalosporins and only needs to be given once a day.

VANCOMYCIN

Vancomycin is a bactericidal antibiotic that is not absorbed orally. It acts by inhibiting peptidoglycan formation and is active against most Gram-positive organisms. Intravenous vancomycin is important for the treatment of patients with septicaemia or endocarditis due to methicillin-resistant strains of *Staphylococcus aureus*. It is the drug of choice (given orally) for antibiotic-associated pseudomembranous colitis (a serious complication of antibiotic therapy caused by a superinfection of the bowel by *Clostridium difficile*, which produces a toxin that damages the colonic mucosa). Rarely, vancomycin may cause renal failure or hearing loss.

‡*Staphylococcus aureas* is a Gram-positive coccus. It is a common cause of infections including boils, wound infections, pneumonia, endocarditis and septicaemia.

39 Antimicrobial drugs that inhibit protein synthesis: aminoglycosides, tetracyclines, macrolides and chloramphenicol

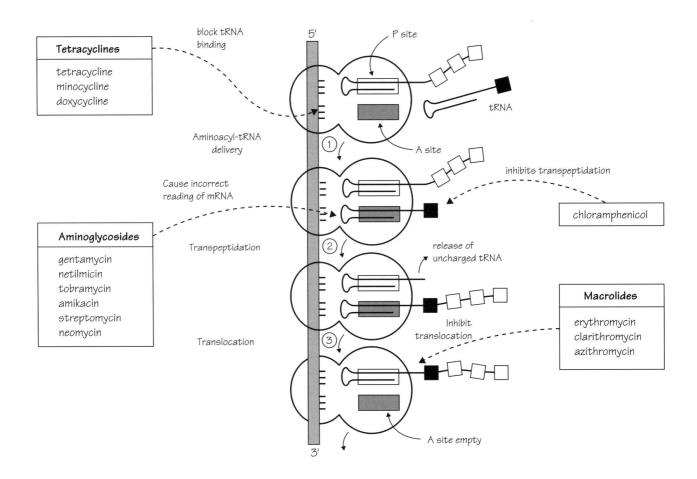

This group of antibiotics acts by inhibiting bacterial protein synthesis. They are selectively toxic because bacterial ribosomes (the sites of protein synthesis) consist of a 50S and a 30S subunit, whilst mammalian ribosomes have a 60S and a 40S subunit.

Proteins are built from amino acids, on ribosomes ( ), which move along (1–2–3) strands of messenger ribonucleic acid (mRNA,) so that successive codons ( ) pass through an acceptor (aminoacyl, A site) for specific transfer RNA (tRNA) molecules that bear the next amino acid (top right,) required to elongate the peptide chain. The **tetracyclines** (top left) and **aminoglycosides** (bottom left) bind to the 30S subunit and *inhibit binding* of the aminoacyl-tRNA. In addition, the aminoglycosides cause *misreading* of mRNA, so that non-functional proteins are synthesized. The next step in peptide synthesis is transpeptidation (2), where the growing peptide chain ( ) attached to the P (peptidyl,) site, is transferred to the amino acid ( ) attached to the aminoacyl-tRNA at the A site. **Chlor-**amphenicol (middle right) *inhibits peptidyl transferase* activity of the 50S ribosomal subunit. Following transpeptidation, the peptide chain is translocated from site A to P (3) so that the A site is ready to accept the next aminoacyl-tRNA. The **macrolides** (bottom right) bind to the 50S subunit and *inhibit translocation*.

The **aminoglycosides**, such as **gentamicin**, must be given by injection. They are valuable drugs in the treatment of severe infections, but are likely to produce nephrotoxic and ototoxic effects. The **tetracyclines** are orally active, wide-spectrum antibiotics, but increasing bacterial resistance has reduced their usefulness. **Macrolides** (e.g. **erythromycin**) have a similar antibacterial spectrum to benzylpenicillin. Gram-positive bacteria are more sensitive to erythromycin than Gram-negative bacteria because they accumulate about 100 times more drug. **Chloramphenicol** is effective against a wide range of organisms, but serious side effects (e.g. aplastic anaemia) restrict its use.

AMINOGLYCOSIDES

The **aminoglycosides** are not absorbed orally and must be given by injection. They are bactericidal but have a narrow therapeutic index and are all potentially toxic. They are excreted by the kidney, and renal impairment results in accumulation and a greater risk of toxic side effects. The most important side effects of the aminoglycosides are damage to the VIIIth cranial nerve (**ototoxicity**) and damage to the **kidneys**. These effects are dose related, and assays of blood aminoglycoside levels should be carried out regularly on all patients receiving aminoglycosides. Aminoglycosides may impair neuromuscular transmission and are therefore contraindicated in patients with myasthenia gravis.

Resistance to aminoglycosides arises from several mechanisms, the most important being the production of enzymes (plasmid controlled) that inactivate the drug by acetylation, phosphorylation or adenylylation. Other mechanisms are the alterations of the envelope to prevent drug access and alteration of the binding site on the 30S subunit so that the drug does not bind (streptomycin only).

Gentamicin is the most important aminoglycoside, its main use being in the 'empirical' treatment of acute life-threatening Gram-negative infections (e.g. *Pseudomonas aeruginosa*) in hospitals, until antibiotic sensitivities are known. Gentamicin may have a synergistic antimicrobial action with penicillin and vancomycin, and combinations with one of these agents are used in the treatment of streptococcal endocarditis. **Amikacin** is less affected by aminoglycoside-inactivating enzymes and is used in serious Gram-negative infections that are gentamicin resistant. **Netilmicin** is claimed to be less toxic than gentamicin. **Streptomycin** is active against *Mycobacterium tuberculosis* and its use is restricted to patients with tuberculosis. It has been largely replaced by rifampicin in combination with other drugs (e.g. isoniazid, pyrazinamide, ethambutol). Streptomycin causes dose-related **ototoxicity**, especially with prolonged or intensive therapy. **Neomycin** is too toxic for parenteral use. It is used topically in skin infections and orally to sterilize the bowel prior to surgery.

MACROLIDES

Macrolides* are usually given orally but **erythromycin** and **clarithromycin** can be given intravenously if necessary. They have a similar antimicrobial spectrum to benzylpenicillin (i.e. narrow spectrum, mainly active against Gram-positive organisms) and can be used as an alternative drug in penicillin-sensitive patients, especially in infections caused by streptococci, staphylococci, pneumococci and clostridia. However, they are ineffective in meningitis because they do not penetrate the central nervous system adequately. Unlike penicillin, the macrolides are effective against several unusual organisms and are specifically indicated in *Mycoplasma* pneumonia and legionnaires' disease. Resistance to macrolides may occur due to plasmid-controlled

*Macrolide: a many-membered lactone ring to which one or more deoxy sugars are attached.

alteration of their receptor on the 50S subunit of the bacterial ribosomes (reducing binding).

Erythromycin is metabolized by the liver and dosage reduction in renal failure is unnecessary unless there is severe failure. The macrolides are very safe drugs. Erythromycin in high doses may cause nausea and vomiting but these effects are less common with azithromycin and clarithromycin. Azithromycin has a very long half-life (40–60 hours) and a single dose is as effective in the treatment of chlamydial non-specific urethritis as tetracyline administered for 7 days. The macrolides inhibit cytochrome P450 and cause accumulation of warfarin, terfenadine and astemizole. High blood levels of these antihistamines can cause hazardous arrhythmias.

TETRACYCLINES

Tetracyclines are usually given orally but may be given by injection. Absorption from the gut is variable and is reduced by calcium ions (milk), magnesium ions (e.g. antacids), food and iron preparations. Tetracyclines are broad-spectrum antibiotics, but there are more suitable agents for most infections. However, they are the drug of choice for treating some infections due to intracellular organisms, because they penetrate macrophages well, e.g. *Chlamydia* (non-specific urethritis, trachoma, psittacosis) and rickettsia (Q-fever). Organisms sensitive to tetracyclines accumulate the drug partly by passive diffusion and partly by active transport. Resistant organisms do not accumulate the antibiotic and selection of microbial populations following the widespread use of tetracyclines in the past has resulted in many resistant strains of streptococci, staphylococci, pneumococci and coliforms. The genes for tetracycline resistance are transmitted by plasmids and are closely associated with those for other drugs to which the organisms will also be resistant (i.e. sulphonamides, aminoglycosides, chloramphenicol). Tetracyclines cause discoloration of the teeth in the young and should be avoided in children up to 8 years of age and in pregnant or lactating women. Diarrhoea and nausea may occur. Overgrowth with *Candida albicans* in the mouth or bowel sometimes leads to thrush.

CHLORAMPHENICOL

Chloramphenicol is given orally or by intravenous injection. It is effective against a wide range of organisms. Unfortunately, serious side effects, which include bone marrow aplasia (incidence about in 40 000—usually fatal), reversible (dose-related) suppression of red and white blood cells, encephalopathy and optic neuritis, restrict its use. Chloramphenicol is indicated in typhoid fever and *Haemophilus influenzae* meningitis. It is metabolized mainly in the liver and penetrates widely, including the brain. Chloramphenicol inhibits the metabolism of other drugs and may potentiate the actions of phenytoin, sulphonylureas and warfarin. Periodic blood counts are required, especially when the drug is given in high doses, for a long time, to patients with renal failure, or to neonates. The latter cannot metabolize the drug rapidly and accumulation causes 'grey baby' syndrome, i.e. pallor, abdominal distension, vomiting and collapse.

40 Antifungal and antiviral drugs

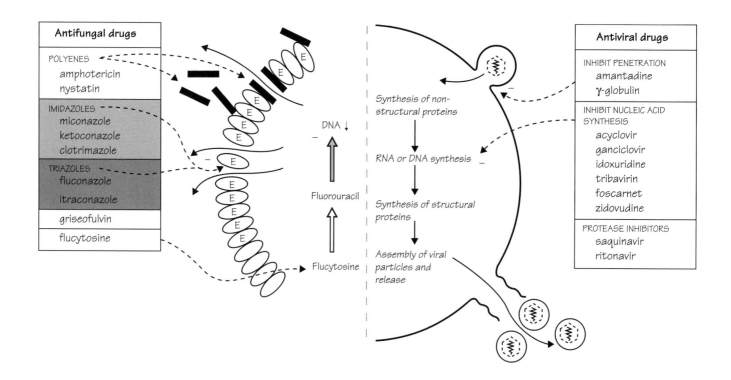

Fungal infections (mycoses) may be superficial or systemic, the latter occurring mostly in immunocompromised patients (acquired immunodeficiency syndrome (AIDS) patients, corticosteroids, anticancer drugs). There are not many effective antifungal drugs (left) and the first-line drug in severe and potentially fatal systemic mycoses, **amphotericin**, is highly toxic. Amphotericin is a polyene antibiotic that interacts (left, ■■■) with ergosterol (E) in the fungal cell membrane and forms pores through which essential fungal cell constituents are lost (⌢➤). The drug is selectively toxic because in human cells the major sterol is cholesterol rather than ergosterol. **Flucytosine** (bottom left) is much less toxic than amphotericin, but its use is limited because it has a narrow spectrum and resistance can develop rapidly during therapy. Flucytosine is converted in fungal cells, but not in human cells, into fluorouracil (⟹) which inhibits DNA synthesis (Chapter 43). The **imidazoles** (left, ▢), which are widely used topically, are broad-spectrum antifungal drugs that act by inhibiting ergosterol synthesis. The **triazoles** (left, ■) are newer drugs, structurally similar to the imidazoles but with a wider range of antifungal activity. They have a lower incidence of adverse effects because they are much more specific inhibitors of lanosterol α-demethylase, action that results in inhibition of ergosterol synthesis. **Griseofulvin** is given orally and is useful for some dermatophyte infections, particularly chronic nail infections. Treatment may need to be prolonged for months. The mechanism of action of griseofulvin may involve interference with microtubule function.

Viruses are intracellular parasites that lack independent metabolism and can replicate only within living host cells. Since their replication cycle is so intimately connected with the metabolic processes of the host cell, it has proved extremely difficult to produce drugs that are selectively toxic to viruses. For this reason, vaccines have been the main method for controlling viral infections (e.g. poliomyelitis, rabies, yellow fever, measles, mumps, rubella). Some effective antiviral drugs (right) have been produced and although they are of limited use, they have transformed the treatment of several diseases, notably those caused by herpes virus infections. Viral replication involves several steps (right figure). **Amantadine** and γ-**globulin** (top right) inhibit penetration of the cell by the virus (⬡), but most antiviral drugs (centre right) are **nucleoside analogues** that interfere with viral (and often human) nucleic acid synthesis. Newer drugs, especially **acyclovir**, which is the most useful agent, are more selectively antiviral, because they are inactive until phosphorylated by enzymes that are preferentially synthesized by the virus. **Zidovudine**, **didanosine** and **zalcitabine** are toxic drugs used only in the treatment of AIDS. Tolerance develops to these drugs and there is an urgent need for more effective agents. In the replication of human immunodeficiency virus (HIV), polypeptide precursors are converted to essential mature proteins (e.g. reverse transcriptase) by a protease. Inhibitors of 'HIV protease' (bottom right) strikingly reduce HIV replication *in vitro* and in combination with other agents (e.g. zidovudine) are currently giving very encouraging results in the treatment of AIDS. **Interferon-α** is an antiviral protein that is normally produced by leucocytes, but can now be obtained by recombinant DNA technology. It is given by intramuscular injection in the treatment of chronic persistent hepatitis B and C.

FUNGAL INFECTIONS

There are three main groups of fungi that cause disease in humans.

1 Moulds (filamentous fungi) grow as long filaments that intertwine to form a mycelium. Examples are the *dermatophytes*, so called because of their ability to digest keratin, which cause infections of the skin, nails and hair, and *Aspergillus fumigatus*, which may cause pulmonary or disseminated aspergillosis.

2 True yeasts are unicellular round or oval fungi, e.g. *Cryptococcus neoformans*, which may cause cryptococcal meningitis or pulmonary infections, usually only in immunocompromised patients.

3 Yeast-like fungi are similar to yeasts but may also form long non-branching filaments. An important example is *Candida albicans*, which is a common commensal organism in the gut, mouth and vagina. It causes a wide range of diseases including oral thrush, vaginitis, endocarditis and septicaemia (often fatal).

POLYENES

Amphotericin is a wide-spectrum antifungal drug used to treat potentially fatal systemic infections due to aspergillus, candida or cryptococcus. It is poorly absorbed orally and is given by intravenous infusion, or intrathecally, when the central nervous system is involved. Adverse effects are very common and most patients develop fever, chills and nausea. Long-term therapy almost inevitably causes renal damage, which is reversible only if detected early. Amphotericin formulated in liposomes is somewhat less toxic. **Nystatin** is too toxic for parenteral use. It is mainly used for *Candida albicans* infections of the skin (cream or ointment) and mucous membranes (tablets sucked in the mouth, vaginal pessaries). Oropharyngeal candidiasis (thrush) is one of the most common features of AIDS and is sometimes a sequel to the use of broad-spectrum antibiotics, anticancer drugs or corticosteroids.

FLUCYTOSINE

Flucytosine is given orally or by intravenous infusion. It is active only against yeasts and is used mainly to treat systemic candidiasis or cryptococcal infections. As resistance often develops rapidly, flucytosine may be given in combination with amphotericin. The drugs act synergistically and the combination is effective in cryptococcal meningitis.

IMIDAZOLES

Imidazoles are wide-spectrum antifungal drugs to which resistance rarely develops. Except for ketoconazole the imidazoles are poorly absorbed orally. **Clotrimazole**, **econazole** and **miconazole** are widely used topically in the treatment of dermatophyte and *Candida albicans* infections. **Miconazole** is used intravenously in systemic infections in patients who cannot tolerate amphotericin. It may cause nausea and vomiting, faintness and anaphylaxis. **Ketoconazole** is well absorbed orally, and has been used in the treatment of local and systemic mycoses. Enthusiasm for ketoconazole has declined because it may cause hepatic necrosis and adrenal suppression.

TRIAZOLES

Fluconazole may be given orally or intravenously and has been successfully used in a wide range of superficial and systemic mycoses (not *Aspergillus*). Unlike ketoconazole, it is not hepatotoxic and does not inhibit adrenal steroid synthesis. **Itraconazole** is absorbed orally and unlike the imidazoles and fluconazole, it is active against *Aspergillus*.

ANTIVIRAL DRUGS

Drugs that stop the virus entering the host cells

Amantadine is given and has been used rather unenthusiastically for the prophylaxis of influenza A infections. The major drawbacks are its narrow spectrum and the fact that influenza vaccine is often preferable.

γ-Globulin. Human immunoglobulin contains specific antibodies against superficial antigens of viruses and can interfere with their entry into the host cells. Normal immunoglobulin injections are used to give temporary protection against hepatitis A.

Drugs that inhibit nucleic acid synthesis

Acyclovir (acycloguanosine). The herpes viruses, e.g. *Herpes simplex* (HSV) and *Varicella zoster* (VZV), contain a thymidine kinase that converts acyclovir to a monophosphate. The monophosphate is subsequently phosphorylated by host cell enzymes to acycloguanosine triphosphate, which inhibits viral DNA polymerase and viral DNA synthesis. Acyclovir is selectively toxic because the thymidine kinase of uninfected host cells activates only a little of the drug, and the DNA polymerase of herpes virus has a much higher affinity for the activated drug than the cellular DNA polymerase. Acyclovir is active against herpes viruses but does not eradicate them. It is effective topically, orally and parenterally, and the appropriate route depends on the site and severity of the infection. Acyclovir is widely used in the treatment of HSV genital infections and high oral doses are effective in treating severe shingles, a painful condition caused by reactivation of a previous infection with VZV (i.e. chickenpox). **Idoxuridine** is also active against HSV but it is too toxic, except for topical use in severe herpetic infections of the skin, eyes and external genitalia. Other drugs have largely superseded idoxuridine.

Ganciclovir must be given intravenously and, because of its toxicity (neutropenia), it is used only to treat severe cytomegalovirus (CMV) infections in immunocompromised patients. CMV is resistant to acyclovir because it does not code for thymidine kinase.

Tribavirin (ribavirin) has been shown to be effective in Lassa fever, a serious arenavirus infection.

Zidovudine (3-azido-3-deoxythymidine) inhibits HIV and is used orally in the treatment of AIDS. The drug is activated by triple phosphorylation and then binds to reverse transcriptase, for which it has 100 times the affinity that it has for cellular DNA polymerases. The drug is incorporated into the DNA chain and because it lacks a 3′ hydroxyl, another nucleotide cannot form a 3′–5′ phosphodiester bond and so the DNA chain is terminated. Resistance develops over 12–18 months and some patients cannot tolerate the severe side effects, which include anaemia, neutropenia, nausea and headaches.

Didanosine (DDL) and **zalcitabine** (DDC) are newer reverse transcriptase inhibitors used in patients with AIDS.

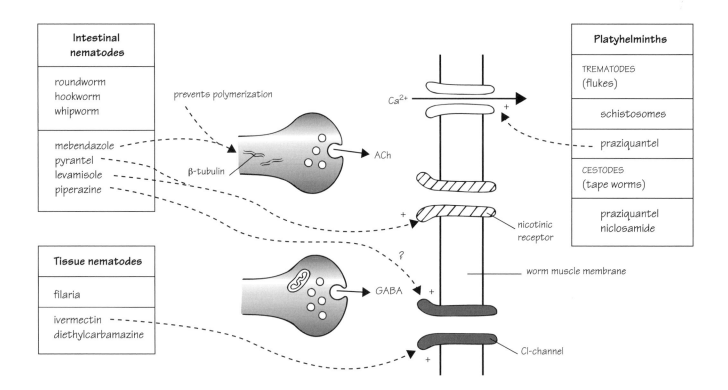

Parasitism is a relationship where one biological species lives in a dependent association with another. Although micro-organisms such as bacteria may be considered to be in such a relationship, only the **protozoa** and **helminths** are generally referred to as parasites. They typically are eukaryotic and have complex life cycles. Only a few parasitic diseases are common in Great Britain (e.g. threadworms, giardiasis; Chapter 42), but in tropical and subtropical areas, where abundant water and high temperatures provide an optimal environment for the larvae and intermediate vector hosts (e.g. mosquitoes), parasitic diseases are common and widespread. Overcrowding, malnutrition and lack of sanitation facilitate the spread of disease and as many as 1000 million people may be infected with parasites. Drugs play an important role in the treatment and control of parasitic diseases but other methods, e.g. vector control by insecticides and land drainage, are also important.

The **helminths** are worms that are round (**nematodes**) (left) or flat (**platyhelminths**) (right). The flat worms are divided into tapeworms (**cestodes**) (bottom right) and flukes (**trematodes**) (top right). The *nervous system* in helminths has important differences from that in vertebrates and these form the basis of the selective toxicity of most drugs used to treat infections with worms (**anthelmintics**). Nematode muscles have both excitatory and inhibitory neuromuscular junctions, the transmitters being acetylcholine (ganglion type nicotinic receptors) and γ-aminobutyric acid (GABA), respectively. **Pyrantel** and **levamisole** (centre left) stimulate the nicotinic receptors and cause a spastic paralysis that results in the worms being expelled. **Ivermectin** (bottom left), a new drug effective against most nematodes, may enhance GABA-mediated inhibition at the neuromuscular junction, whilst **piperazine** (centre left) may act as a GABA agonist. Both drugs cause flaccid paralysis of the worms. GABAergic drugs are ineffective against trematodes and cestodes because they do not have peripheral GABAergic nerves. **Praziquantel** (right), a highly effective agent, induces muscular contraction and spastic paralysis in these parasites by increasing calcium fluxes. Some anthelmintics have quite well-characterized biochemical actions. In particular, the benzimidazole derivatives, e.g. **mebendazole** (centre left), bind to β-tubulin in nematode cells with a much higher affinity than they do to human tubulin, and block the transport of secretory granules and other organelles. The mechanism of action of some anthelmintics is unknown, e.g. **diethylcarbamazine**, a drug used in the treatment of lymphatic filariasis.

NEMATODES (ROUNDWORMS)

Ascaris lumbricoides (common roundworm) infects the gut lumen in about 25% of the world's population. The worms, which are between 10 and 30 cm long, are common in the subtropics, especially in areas where sanitation is poor. Treatment is with oral **mebendazole, levamisole** or **pyrantel**. **Piperazine** is also effective but may cause vomiting and diarrhoea.

Hookworm is infection of the gut with either *Ancylostoma duodenale* or *Necator americanus*. These small worms (about 1 cm long) grip the mucosa and take a little blood from the host each day. Hookworm is a common cause of iron deficiency anaemia in tropical and subtropical countries. **Mebendazole** and **pyrantel** are effective.

Strongyloidiasis infects the gut, but many people infected with these small worms (2 mm long) are asymptomatic. Treatment is with **thiabendazole** or **albendazole**.

Threadworms (pinworm). Infection with *Enterobius vermicularis* (about 1 cm long) is very common, especially in children. Pruritis ani is the main symptom. Female worms deposit eggs on the perianal skin and this causes irritation. The lava are often reingested via the fingers and this maintains a cycle of autoinfection. The whole family is usually treated with **mebendazole** or **pyrantel** which are highly effective.

Whipworms. *Trichuris trichiauria* causes infection of the gut lumen, often together with *Ascaris* and hookworms. Light asymptomatic infection is common. **Mebendazole** is effective but pyrantel is not.

Filarial infections. Both the adult and larval (microfilariae) forms of the filariae occur in humans. Transmission is by the bite of blood-sucking insects. The adult worms are very long-lived and the shedding of microfilariae lasts for many years. The severity of the disease depends on the adult worm burden of the host.

Lymphatic filariasis is infection, usually with *Wuchereria bancrofti*, *Brugia malayi* or *B. timori*, caused by the bite of mosquito vectors. Adult worms living in the lymphatic vessels cause pathological changes that may result in obstructive lymphodema. About 90 million people are infected, two-thirds of them living in China, India and Indonesia. **Onchocerciasis** is infection with *Onchocerca volvulus* and occurs mainly in tropical Africa and central America. Transmission is by the Simulium blackfly. Most human infections are acquired near rivers because these are required by the blackfly to breed. Death of the microfilariae in the skin causes chronic pruritis, and in the cornea eventually causes scarring and blindness (river blindness).

Diethylcarbamazine and ivermectin are used in filarial infections. The treatment of onchocerciasis was for many years with **diethylcarbamazine** which kills microfiliariae (by an unknown mechanism) but not adult worms. Unfortunately, killing the microfiliariae exacerbates the disease, often with severe reactions where there are lesions in the eyes. **Ivermectin** causes much less exacerbation of the disease and is now the treatment of choice.

Toxocariasis is caused by infection with larval forms of *Toxocara canis* or *T. cati*. Eggs shed in the faeces of dogs and cats are ingested (most often by children) and release larvae, which become disseminated to many organs including the eye. Dead worms evoke granuloma formation and may cause blindness. Treatment is with **diethylcarbamazine** which kills migrating worms but cannot affect fibrosing lesions already present.

TREMATODES (FLUKES)

Schistosomiasis (bilharziasis) is infection with flukes of the genus *Schistosoma*; these flukes affect the bladder and urinary tract (*S. haematobium*) or intestine (*S. mansoni*, *S. japonicum*). The secondary host is an aquatic snail that releases cercariae into the water. Children are infected early in life by playing in infected water. Treatment is with **praziquantel**, which is effective in all fluke infections (except the liver fluke *Fasciola hepatica*).

CESTODES (TAPE WORMS)

Taenia saginata and *T. solium* infections occur after eating undercooked infected beef and pork, respectively. The scolex evaginates from the ingested cysticercus (larval stage) and fixes to the gut wall. Then, self-fertile proglottids develop. The worm may be 5–10 m long but often causes no symptoms. Fish tapeworm (*Diphyllobrothrium latum*) infection is obtained by eating infected uncooked fish. **Praziquantel** is effective in tapeworm infections.

ANTHELMINTICS

Mebendazole and albendazole are benzimidazoles given orally. They have a wide range of action, especially against intestinal nematodes. Mebendazole and albendazole have few side effects, probably because they have low systemic bioavailability.

Pyrantel is a depolarizing neuromuscular blocking drug and anticholinesterase that produces a spastic paralysis in hookworms, pinworms and roundworms. The drug is given orally and is selectively toxic because little is absorbed from the gut. Side effects include mild gastrointestinal upsets. **Levamisole** has similar actions as those of pyrantel and is very effective in roundworm infections.

Ivermectin binds to invertebrate GABA receptors with an affinity about 100 times greater than that for vertebrate receptors and may paralyse the worms by increasing GABA-mediated inhibition. However, recent studies suggest that ivermectin activates a glutamate-gated chloride channel found only in invertebrates. Cestodes and trematodes lack high-affinity binding sites for ivermectin and so the drug is ineffective against these helminths. Ivermectin is active against the microfilariae of *Onchocerca volvulus* but not the adult worm. It is also highly effective against ascariasis, enterobiasis, trichuriasis and strongyloidiasis. Ivermectin is given orally and has few side effects. A single dose of the drug given every 6–12 months controls, but does not cure, onchocerciasis.

Praziquantel is given orally and has no serious unwanted effects. It is highly effective against many trematodes and cestodes (but not nematodes). The drug is taken up by susceptible helminths and increases membrane permeability to calcium. This causes a spastic paralysis and detachment of the worms. Perhaps more importantly, praziquantel damages the tegmentum, causing activation of host defence mechanisms and destruction of the helminths.

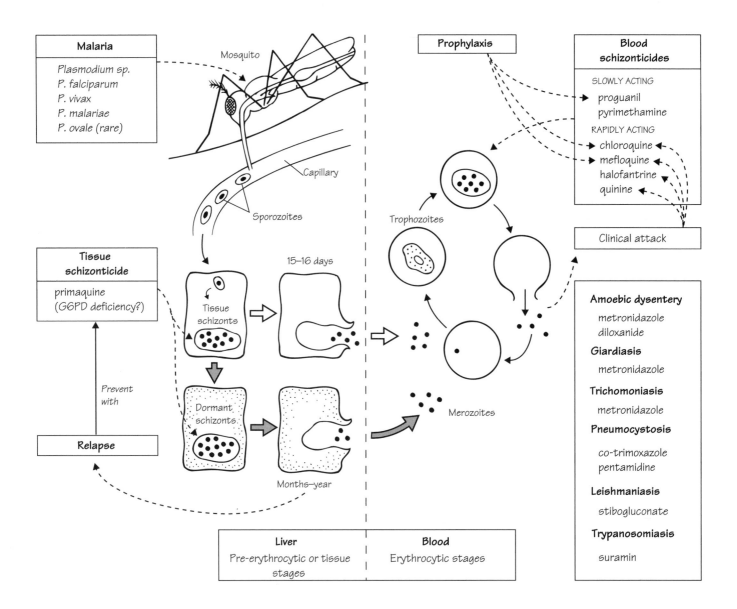

Malaria is the most serious protozoal disease and although it is not endemic in Europe or North America, travellers to malarial areas risk infection. This risk can be greatly reduced by taking prophylactic drugs (prophylaxis, top right) but drug-resistant *Plasmodium falciparum* is an increasing problem in many parts of the world and travellers are at increased risk of this potentially life-threatening form of malaria. There is no prophylactic drug treatment for other protozoal infections (right bottom) and some, e.g. giardiasis, are quite common.

Malaria is caused by four species of protozoa (top left) that have part of their life cycle in the female *Anopheles* mosquito. When a mosquito bites a human, it injects sporozoites into a capillary (⬬) (top left of figure) and these are carried in the blood to the liver, where they multiply and form tissue schizonts. This is the pre-erythrocytic or primary tissue stage of the disease (left half of the figure). After 5–16 days the schizonts rupture and release (⟹) thousands of merozoites (●)

which infect red blood cells (◯) and start the erythrocytic stage of the disease (right figure). In the case of *P. vivax* and *P. ovale* (but not *P. falciparum*) some of the schizonts in the liver remain dormant (▱) and these may rupture months or years later, causing a relapse of the disease (⟹).

Most antimalarials are toxic to the erythrocytic schizonts (blood schizonticides, top right) and the rapidly acting ones (**chloroquine, quinine, mefloquine** and **halofantrine**) are used to treat clinical attacks of malaria. **Proguanil** acts too slowly for this purpose and is used to provide prophylaxis. Chloroquine and mefloquine are used for both prophylaxis and treatment (quinine is too toxic for prophylaxis). **Primaquine** (left) is a tissue schizonticide used to eliminate the schizonts in the liver (radical cure) once the clinical attack has been controlled with chloroquine or quinine.

BLOOD SCHIZONTICIDES (SLOWLY ACTING)

Proguanil and **pyrimethamine** are effective schizonticides but their action is too slow to treat acute attacks. Proguanil is used, usually with chloroquine, for the prophylaxis of malaria. Pyrimethamine is given in combination with sulphadoxine (Fansidar) following the use of quinine to treat *P. falciparum* infection. Maloprim, a combination of pyrimethamine with dapsone, is sometimes used with chloroquine for prophylaxis where there is a high risk of chloroquine-resistant *P. falciparum*. Sulfadoxine and dapsone act on the same pathway as pyrimethamine, but at a different point (Chapter 37).

Mechanism of action. Pyrimethamine and the active metabolite of proguanil (cycloguanil) are folate antagonists. They inhibit dihydrofolate reductase, and by preventing the regeneration of tetrahydrofolate they inhibit DNA synthesis and cell division. The drugs are selectively toxic because they have 1000 times the affinity for the plasmodial enzyme than for the human enzyme (compare with methotrexate (Chapter 43), which has a high affinity for the human enzyme).

BLOOD SCHIZONTICIDES (RAPIDLY ACTING)

Chloroquine usually controls the fever of malaria within 24–48 hours. It is used to treat *P. vivax* and *P. ovale* infections but it has no action on the liver schizonts and must be followed by a course of primaquine. In most areas of the world *P. falciparum* has become resistant to the drug, which should not be used for treatment. Chloroquine is usually given orally but may be given by intravenous infusion to seriously ill patients.

Mechanism of action. Plasmodia within parasitized erythrocytes digest haemoglobin, producing haem (ferriprotoporphyrin IX) which is toxic. Plasmodial haem polymerase converts haem to harmless haemazoin. Chloroquine (and quinine) is concentrated in sensitive plasmodia and inhibits haem polymerase. The resulting accumulation of haem is thought to kill the parasites by a membranolytic action.

Adverse effects. These are unusual with the low doses used for prophylaxis. The higher doses used for treatment may cause nausea, vomiting, diarrhoea, rashes, pruritis and, rarely, psychoses. Prolonged administration of high doses may irreversibly damage the retina.

Quinine, **mefloquine** and **halofantrine** are used orally to treat *P. falciparum* infections (malignant tertian malaria). Quinine can be given by intravenous infusion if necessary (e.g. unconsciousness). A 7-day course of quinine is given. If quinine resistance is known or suspected, it is followed by Fansidar or tetracycline (if Fansidar resistant). Combined therapy is not necessary with mefloquine or halofantrine, which are more potent and less toxic than quinine.

Adverse effects of quinine include abdominal pain, nausea, tinnitus, headache, blindness and hypersensitivity reactions. Mefloquine may cause neuropsychiatric reactions. The mechanisms of action of quinine, mefloquine and halofantrine are unknown.

TISSUE SCHIZONTICIDE

Primaquine is an important drug because it is the only antimalarial that will kill the schizonts of *P. vivax* and *P. ovale* lying dormant in the liver. However, it is of no value in treating clinical attacks because it has lit-

tle effect on the erythrocytic schizonts. The mechanism of action of primaquine is unknown. It seems that oxidative damage to the parasite is caused by active metabolites that may also cause haemolysis of erythrocytes in persons with an inherited deficiency of glucose-6-phosphate dehydrogenase (G6PD). For this reason, the blood of patients should be tested for G6PD activity before starting treatment with primaquine.

Adverse effects include nausea, vomiting, bone marrow depression and haemolytic anaemia.

AMOEBIC DYSENTERY

Amoebiasis is caused by infection with *Entamoeba histolytica*. **Metronidazole** (Chapter 37) is used in acute infections but in asymptomatic infections, where cysts are present, diloxanide furoate is also necessary.

GIARDIASIS

Giardia lamblia is a flagellate pear-shaped protozoon. It is a common bowel pathogen causing flatulence and diarrhoea. Metronidazole is effective.

TRICHOMONIASIS

Trichomonas vaginalis is a common cause of vaginal discharge and occasionally causes urethritis in both sexes. **Metronidazole** is usually very effective.

PNEUMOCYSTOSIS

Pneumocystis carinii is a common organism that is probably inhaled in early life and lies dormant in the lungs. In immunosuppressed patients (steroids, immunosuppressive drugs, AIDS) it may cause an interstitial pneumonitis. *P. carinii* pneumonia is the most common presentation of AIDS in Western countries. It is treated with **co-trimoxazole** (Chapter 37) or **pentamidine** given parenterally or by inhalation. The mechanism of action of pentamidine is unknown. It has many side effects which are sometimes fatal.

LEISHMANIASIS

The *Leishmania* are intracellular protozoan parasites that are transmitted to humans by the bite of infected sandflies. Both cutaneous leishmaniasis and visceral leishmaniasis (kala-azar) are treated with **stibogluconate**, an organic pentavalent antimony compound that reacts with thiol groups and reduces ATP production in the parasite. **Pentamidine** and **amphotericin** (Chapter 40) are second-line drugs.

TRYPANOSOMIASIS

African trypanosomiasis (sleeping sickness) is spread by the tsetse fly and is due to infection with either *Trypanosoma gambiense* or *T. rhodesiense*. **Suramin** kills the parasites in blood and lymphoid nodes by an unknown mechanism and is curative early in the disease. It does not cross the blood–brain barrier and is ineffective when there is neurological involvement.

43 Drugs used in cancer

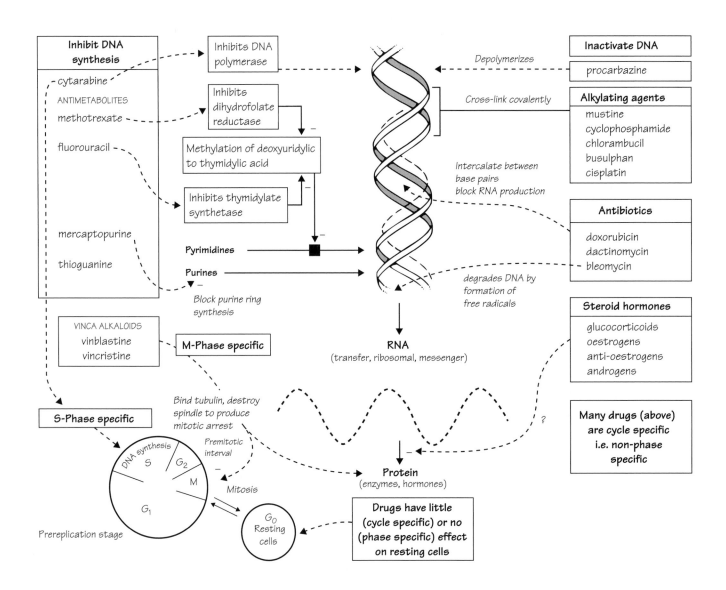

The aim of treatment in patients with cancer is cure, or if this is not possible, effective palliation. Many cancers present as localized tumour masses, but surgery or radiotherapy often fail to eradicate the disease, which eventually becomes widespread. For this reason, there is a trend to incorporate systemic treatment with local treatment at the time of diagnosis.

Drugs used to treat cancer inhibit the mechanisms of cell proliferation. They are therefore toxic to both tumour cells and proliferating normal cells, especially in the *bone marrow, gastrointestinal epithelium* and *hair follicles*. The **selectivity** of cytotoxic drugs occurs because in malignant tumours a higher proportion of the component cells is undergoing division than in normal proliferating tissues.

Anticancer drugs are classified according to their sites of action along the synthetic pathway of cellular macromolecules (top). Some drugs are only effective during part of the cell cycle (**phase-specific drugs**, left), whilst others (**cycle-specific drugs**, right) are cytotoxic throughout the cell cycle (lower figure).

Alkylating agents (top right) readily form covalent bonds. They

react with the bases in DNA and prevent cell division by cross-linking the two strands of the double helix. Several **antibiotics** (middle right) isolated from various species of *Streptomyces* also interact with DNA and are widely used as anticancer drugs. Some cytotoxic drugs act by interfering with DNA synthesis (top left). These agents are **antimetabolites** and inhibit purine or pyrimidine synthesis. One is a folic acid antagonist (methotrexate). The **vinca alkaloids** (bottom left) inhibit mitosis by binding to the microtubular proteins necessary for spindle formation. A miscellaneous group of drugs is also used in the treatment of cancer, e.g. procarbazine. **Steroid hormones** and hormone antagonists (lower right) are often used in the treatment of cancer. **Combinations** of cytotoxic drugs may be strikingly more successful than single drugs in the treatment of some cancers (e.g. Hodgkin's disease).

The administration of cytotoxic drugs may be associated with unpleasant and even life-threatening **adverse effects**. Individual drugs sometimes have specific toxic effects, but general adverse effects common to many agents include nausea and vomiting (reduced by antiemetics such as prochlorperazine, dexamethasone and ondansetron), oral and intestinal ulceration, diarrhoea, alopecia and bone marrow suppression, which can decrease production of any or all of the formed elements of blood. Leucopenia is associated with an increased risk of opportunistic infections; thrombocytopenia leads to bleeding, and decreased red cell formation causes anaemia. *Vincristine* and *bleomycin* are exceptions that do not cause myelosuppression.

DRUG COMBINATIONS

The administration of combinations of drugs given intermittently often produces better results than more continuous treatment with a single drug. The rationale is that a combination of drugs with different toxic effects and affecting different biochemical pathways has higher antitumour activity without additive toxicity. For example, the combination of mustine, vincristine, procarbazine and prednisone (MOPP) induces remission in 80% of patients with Hodgkin's disease, whilst the drugs used individually induce remission in less than 40% of patients.

SELECTIVITY

The selectivity of antitumour drugs is marginal at best. Their beneficial effects depend on the bone marrow cells recovering faster than the tumour cells after drug administration. Following marrow recovery, more drug can be given, and because a fixed proportion of tumour cells are killed during each period of drug administration, the tumour may eventually be eradicated. In practice, the response of tumours to chemotherapy ranges from 'cure', e.g. acute lymphoblastic leukaemia in children, to being completely refractory, e.g. colorectal carcinoma.

ALKYLATING AGENTS

These drugs are widely used in cancer chemotherapy. Prolonged usage often affects gametogenesis severely; most males become permanently sterile. The drugs are associated with an increased incidence of acute non-lymphocytic leukaemia. **Cyclophosphamide** is metabolized in the liver, forming several active metabolites. One metabolite, acrolein, occasionally causes haemorrhagic cystitis, a serious complication. Intravenous 2-*m*ercapto*e*thane *s*ulphonate sodium (*Na*) (mesna) protects the bladder by combining with acrolein in the kidney. Cyclophosphamide is extensively used in a wide variety of cancers, usually in combination with other drugs. **Chlorambucil** is given orally. It is tending to replace other alkylating agents because it has milder adverse effects. **Mustine** is given intravenously in Hodgkin's disease. It is very toxic and causes severe vomiting.

CYTOTOXIC ANTIBIOTICS

Doxorubicin is one of the most successful antitumour drugs and is used in acute leukaemias, lymphomas and a variety of solid tumours. Doxorubicin is an anthracycline that can slip between neighbouring base pairs in DNA (intercalation). It inhibits DNA and RNA synthesis, probably by an action on topoisomerase II and/or by the production of free radicals. High cumulative doses are cardiotoxic, probably because oxygen free radicals are formed; these are not inactivated in the heart because it lacks catalase.

VINCA ALKALOIDS

Vincristine is used in acute lymphoblastic leukaemia, lymphomas and some solid tumours. It has toxic effects on peripheral and autonomic nerves. **Vinblastine** is used in the treatment of lymphomas and testicular teratomas. It causes more myelosuppression than vincristine but is less neurotoxic.

ANTIMETABOLITES

Folic acid antagonists. Methotrexate competitively inhibits dihydrofolate reductase and prevents the regeneration of tetrahydrofolic acid and the co-enzyme, methylene tetrahydrofolate, which is essential for the conversion of deoxyuridylic acid to thymidylic acid. Since rapidly dividing cells require an abundant supply of deoxythymidylate for the synthesis of DNA, methotrexate prevents the division of cells. It is used in acute lymphatic leukaemia, lymphomas and several solid tumours.

Antipyrimidines. Fluorouracil is converted to fluorodeoxyuridylic acid, which inhibits thymidylate synthetase, the enzyme responsible for converting deoxyuridylate to thymidylic acid. This impairs DNA synthesis by reducing the availability of thymidylic acid. It is mainly given intravenously and is used in the treatment of solid tumours, especially breast cancer. It is the drug of choice for metastatic colon cancer. **Cytarabine** is used in acute leukaemia and lymphomas.

Antipurines impair the synthesis of purine nucleotides but the mechanisms involved are not clear. **Mercaptopurine** is used for maintenance therapy in patients with acute leukaemias.

HORMONES

Glucocorticoids (e.g. **prednisolone**) inhibit cell division by interfering with DNA synthesis. They are widely used in the treatment of leukaemias, lymphomas and breast cancer. **Sex hormones and antagonists.** The growth of some tumours, especially carcinoma of the breast and prostate, is partly dependent upon hormones. Removal of the gland producing the hormone (e.g. orchidectomy in prostatic cancer), the administration of hormones with the opposite action or the administration of an antagonist may induce tumour regression. **Tamoxifen**, an oestrogen antagonist, is widely used in the treatment of postmenopausal metastatic breast cancer. In prostatic cancer, **stilboestrol** has been replaced by gonadotrophin-releasing hormone (GnRH) analogues (e.g. **buserelin**) which have fewer adverse affects. When given continuously GnRH analogues paradoxically inhibit luteinizing hormone (LH) secretion, thereby suppressing testosterone release. Unfortunately, the effects of hormones are usually temporary, because hormone-independent cells eventually predominate.

Immunosuppressants are used to prevent tissue rejection after organ transplantation, and to treat autoimmune and collagen diseases. **Azathioprine** is converted to mercaptopurine in the body and is widely used in combination with **prednisolone**. The glucocorticoids act mainly on polymorph and macrophage activity. **Cyclosporin** is a potent immunosuppressant used especially to prevent rejection of organ and tissue transplants. It is not myelotoxic but may cause kidney damage.

44 Poisoning

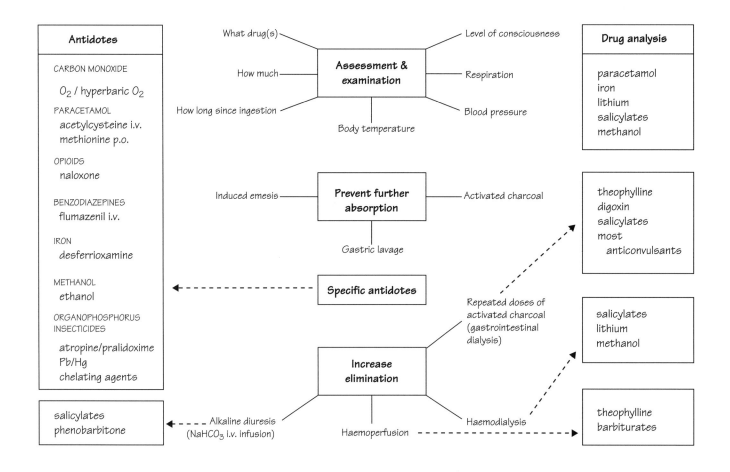

Antidotes

CARBON MONOXIDE
O_2 / hyperbaric O_2

PARACETAMOL
acetylcysteine i.v.
methionine p.o.

OPIOIDS
naloxone

BENZODIAZEPINES
flumazenil i.v.

IRON
desferrioxamine

METHANOL
ethanol

ORGANOPHOSPHORUS INSECTICIDES
atropine/pralidoxime
Pb/Hg
chelating agents

salicylates
phenobarbitone

What drug(s) — How much — How long since ingestion — **Assessment & examination** — Level of consciousness — Respiration — Blood pressure — Body temperature

Drug analysis

paracetamol
iron
lithium
salicylates
methanol

Induced emesis — **Prevent further absorption** — Activated charcoal

Gastric lavage

Specific antidotes

Repeated doses of activated charcoal (gastrointestinal dialysis)

theophylline
digoxin
salicylates
most anticonvulsants

salicylates
lithium
methanol

Increase elimination

Alkaline diuresis ($NaHCO_3$ i.v. infusion) — Haemoperfusion — Haemodialysis

theophylline
barbiturates

The commonest drugs causing death by self-poisoning are **Co-prox-amol**,* **paracetamol** alone, and **tricyclic antidepressants**. However, the commonest cause of fatal self-poisoning, especially in men, is **carbon monoxide** originating from a car exhaust. Self-poisoning with two or more drugs is not uncommon and alcohol is also taken in about 50% of incidents. Most cases of intentional self-poisoning are cries for help (parasuicide) but over 3000 people a year successfully kill themselves by poisoning. Once in hospital the mortality of self-poisoners is less than 1%. Accidental self-poisoning occurs mainly in young children (under 5 years) and usually involves medicines or household chemicals (e.g. bleach) left within reach. Patients presenting with poisoning must be given an initial assessment (top) including a rapid but careful clinical examination. It is important to exclude other causes of coma and abnormal behaviour (e.g. head injury, epilepsy, diabetes). Most patients admitted for self-poisoning require only **general supportive measures**. Drug screens are rarely needed as an emergency, but with some drugs (top right) the clinical state of the patient may not reflect the severity of the overdose and measurement of the plasma concentration can indicate the use of life-saving techniques (centre bottom) or **specific antidotes** (left).

Further absorption of the drug can be reduced either by causing emesis with **syrup of ipecacuanha** (conscious patients only) or by **gastric aspiration and lavage**. The sooner after drug ingestion the stomach is washed out, the more drug is likely to be recovered. Gastric lavage is commonly performed up to 4 hours after drug ingestion, but may be worthwhile up to 10 hours after tricyclics (and other drugs that slow gastric emptying) and up to 24 hours after aspirin ingestion. Increasingly, the oral administration of **activated charcoal** is being used to reduce drug absorption. Techniques used to **increase drug elimination** (bottom) have a limited role, but are important in severely poisoned patients.

*Paracetamol + dextropropoxyphene.

REDUCTION OF ABSORPTION

Emesis. Syrup of ipecacuanha induces emesis in over 90% of patients within 30 minutes. It can only be used in conscious patients and is preferred in children because gastric lavage is unpleasant.

Gastric aspiration and lavage is more effective than emesis and is the only option in unconscious patients. An orogastric tube is passed into the stomach, which is then washed out with 300–600 ml of water (three or four times). If the patient is unconscious the airway must be protected with a cuffed endotracheal tube. Activated charcoal (50 g) is left in the stomach unless an oral antidote is to be given (charcoal will absorb antidote as well as drug). Gastric lavage and induced emesis are contraindicated in poisoning with corrosives or petroleum compounds.

Activated charcoal is a very fine porous black powder with an enormous surface area in relation to weight ($1000 \, m^2 \, g^{-1}$). It binds many drugs and 10 g of charcoal will absorb about 1 g of drug. Charcoal does not absorb iron, lithium, corrosive agents or organic solvents.

ENHANCEMENT OF ELIMINATION

Enhancement of elimination can reduce the time of recovery but there is little evidence that it changes morbidity, except in severely comatose patients (grade IV coma).

Repeated doses of activated charcoal. Repeated oral doses of charcoal may increase elimination by gastrointestinal dialysis; it has the merit of being very safe (unless aspirated).

Alkaline diuresis. The urine is made alkaline (pH 7.5–8.5) by the administration of $NaHCO_3$ (intravenous infusion) This ionizes weak acids, e.g. aspirin, in the renal tubules and reduces reabsorption. Similarly, acid diuresis may be useful in cases of poisoning with basic drugs such as amphetamine and ecstasy. Forced alkaline diuresis using large intravenous volumes of water containing $NaHCO_3$ is hazardous and no longer recommended.

Haemodialysis and haemoperfusion are invasive techniques requiring cannulation of an artery and vein (usually in the arm) to establish a temporary extra-corporeal circulation. In haemodialysis the drug passes down its concentration gradient through the dialysis membrane and is removed in the dialysis fluid. In haemoperfusion the blood is passed through a column of activated charcoal or resin onto which the drug is absorbed. These techniques have significant risks (haemorrhage, air embolism, infection, loss of a peripheral artery).

ASPIRIN

The symptoms of salicylate poisoning include tinnitis, hyperventilation and sweating. Coma is uncommon and indicates very severe poisoning. Acid–base disturbances are complicated because aspirin stimulates the respiratory centre, causing a respiratory alkalosis, but also uncouples oxidative phosphorylation, which may cause a metabolic acidosis. Immediate management includes measurement of plasma salicylate concentration, electrolytes and blood gases. Gastric lavage is worth-

while up to 24 hours after ingestion, followed by activated charcoal administration. Severe poisoning (plasma concentration above $500 \, mg \, l^{-1}$) requires urinary alkalinization. In very severe poisoning haemodialysis is the treatment of choice.

PARACETAMOL

Patients may be asymptomatic or complain only of nausea and vomiting, but after a delay of 48–72 hours relatively small amounts (more than 10 g, 20–30 tablets) may cause fatal hepatocellular necrosis. Normally, paracetamol is metabolized, mainly by conjugation reactions in the liver but high doses saturate these pathways and the drug is then oxidized to a reactive (toxic) quinone intermediate (*N*-acetylbenzoquinoneimine). The quinone can be inactivated by combination with glutathione but high doses of paracetamol deplete the hepatic glutathione stores and the reactive quinone then covalently binds to thiol groups on the cell proteins and kills the cell. **Acetylcysteine** (intravenous or oral) and **methionine** (oral) are potentially life-saving antidotes in cases of paracetamol poisoning because they increase the synthesis of liver glutathione. Patients who have taken an overdose of paracetamol should immediately have a blood sample taken to determine quickly the plasma concentration of drug so that the antidote can be given. If less than 4 hours have elapsed since ingestion, the stomach should be emptied. The decision on whether to continue treatment with the antidote is decided by referring the plasma paracetamol concentration to a nomogram, which joins plots of $200 \, mg \, l^{-1}$ at 4 hours and $30 \, mg \, l^{-1}$ at 15 hours. This nomogram is based on outcome studies of many fatal and non-fatal cases of poisoning carried out before effective treatment became available. If the patient's drug concentration is above this '200-line' then antidote treatment is continued. Patients taking enzyme-inducing drugs (including alcohol) are at increased risk, and for these patients the antidote is given if the plasma concentration of paracetamol is above the '100-line' (joining $100 \, mg \, l^{-1}$ at 4 hours and $15 \, mg \, l^{-1}$ at 15 hours). If the time of ingestion is less than 4 hours the plasma concentration is unreliable because paracetamol absorption will be continuing. The most effective antidote is acetylcysteine given intravenously within 8 hours of paracetamol ingestion. Adverse effects, including anaphylactoid reactions, occur in about 15% of patients.

Opioids cause coma, pin-point pupils and respiratory depression. They are specifically antagonized by **naloxone**, which is given intravenously in repeated doses until ventilation is adequate. Naloxone has a shorter half-life than most opioids and toxicity may recur, necessitating further doses. Naloxone may cause an acute withdrawal syndrome in opioid addicts.

Tricyclic antidepressants

Toxicity following overdosage arises mainly from central anticholinergic effects (respiratory depression, hallucinations, convulsions) and cardiotoxicity. Most patients require only observation or simple supportive measures such as oxygen to correct hypoxia. The commonest arrhythmia is sinus tachycardia due to an atropine-like effect. Lengthening of the QRS complex (a quinidine-like effect) is an ominous sign and may presage convulsions, which may be controlled by intravenous **diazepam** or **chlormethiazole**.

45 Adverse drug reactions

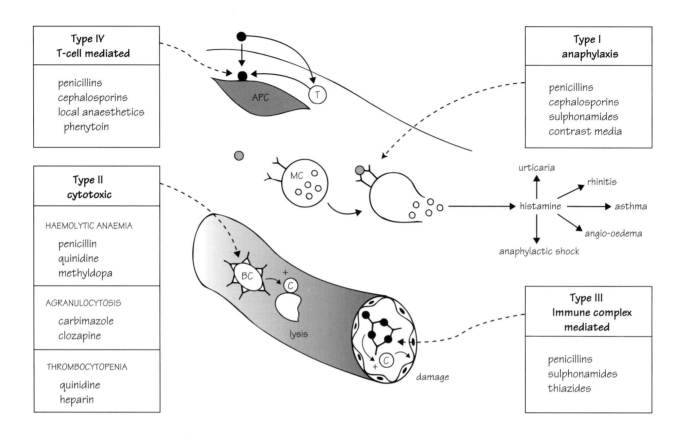

The incidence of adverse (harmful) drug reactions is difficult to establish but up to 5% of acute admissions to hospital result from an adverse reaction to drugs given in general practice. In hospital, up to 20% of patients experience an adverse drug reaction, and although these are rarely life threatening, they account for 0.5–1% of hospital in-patient deaths. The majority of adverse drug reactions can be divided into those that are **dose related** (not illustrated) and those that are **non-dose related**; the latter, which occur infrequently, often have an immunological basis (see figure). A few drugs are associated with an increased incidence of birth defects (**teratogens**) or tumours (**carcinogens**). Some drugs, when given continuously, lead to **adaptive changes**, and stopping the drug causes unwanted withdrawal effects (e.g. benzodiazepines—insomnia and anxiety; corticosteroids—acute adrenal insufficiency).

Dose related (type A) adverse drug reactions are predictable and are caused by an excess of the drug's wanted pharmacological effect (e.g. hypoglycaemia with insulin, bleeding with heparin) or sometimes a drug's parallel unwanted action (e.g. respiratory depression with morphine). Dose related adverse drug reactions occur most often with drugs that have a steep dose–response curve and/or a small difference between therapeutic and toxic doses (i.e. a low **therapeutic index = toxic dose/therapeutic dose**). Commonly used drugs with a **low therapeutic index** include *anticoagulants, hypoglycaemic drugs, digoxin, anti-arrhythmics, aminoglycosides, xanthines, cytotoxic and immunosuppressive drugs.* Dose related adverse drug reactions are usually due to *incorrect dosage* (too high) or *altered pharmacokinetics,* usually impaired drug elimination (e.g. renal failure). **Drug interactions** are involved in 10–20% of adverse drug reactions and are especially common in the elderly, who are more likely to receive multiple drugs for multiple ailments.

Non-dose related (idiosyncratic, type B) adverse drug reactions are relatively rare, but are unpredictable, and in contrast to dose related adverse drug reactions have a considerable mortality. Drug allergy may involve hypersensitivity reactions (types I to IV) (figure) but others are not easily classified. Anaphylaxis is the most common serious drug allergy and is potentially fatal.

DOSE-RELATED (TYPE A) ADVERSE REACTIONS

Pharmacokinetic variations

The elimination of drugs is very variable in normal individuals and genetic factors can reduce drug elimination and cause adverse reactions (e.g. succinylcholine causes prolonged apnoea in patients with defective pseudocholinesterase; Chapter 4). **Renal disease** can lead to accumulation and toxicity if a drug is excreted by glomerular filtration or tubular secretion (e.g. gentamicin and other aminoglycosides, digoxin, amphotericin, captopril).

Drug interactions

Drug interaction is the modification of the action of one drug by another and involves **pharmacodynamic** or **pharmacokinetic** mechanisms. Drugs with steep dose–response curves and serious dose-related toxicities are especially likely to be involved in adverse drug interactions (i.e. those with a low therapeutic index, opposite page).

Pharmacodynamic interactions

Pharmacodynamic interactions are the commonest and usually have a simple mechanism. Thus, drugs with similar actions, e.g. benzodiazepines and alcohol, produce additive effects and may cause severe central nervous system depression. Conversely, drugs may have opposing actions, e.g. in asthmatic patients β-blockers will oppose β-agonists (and theophylline) and may precipitate severe or even fatal asthma.

Pharmacokinetic interactions

Absorption may be affected by drugs that increase (e.g. metoclopramide) or decrease (e.g. atropine) the rate of gastric emptying. Enterohepatic recirculation of oral contraceptives (especially low-dose oestrogen) may be decreased by antibiotics and lead to pregnancy (antibiotics kill the gut bacteria that normally release the steroid from the conjugated form excreted in bile).

Distribution. Many drugs are bound to plasma albumin and may be displaced by a second drug. With the exception of a few drugs (e.g warfarin, phenytoin, tolbutamide), which are more than 90% bound, the displacement of drugs by this mechanism is usually of little practical consequence because increased elimination quickly reduces the plasma concentration of free drug to its original value.

Metabolism. Induction of hepatic enzymes by a second drug (e.g. phenytoin, phenobarbitone, carbamazepine, rifampicin) can decrease the efficacy of drugs metabolized by the same enzymes (e.g. warfarin). Enzyme inhibitors (e.g. cimetidine) potentiate the effects of warfarin and may cause phenytoin and theophylline toxicity. Other examples are discussed in Chapter 4.

Excretion. Drugs may share the same transport system in the proximal tubules. Thus, probenecid competitively reduces penicillin excretion. Thiazide and loop diuretics reduce sodium reabsorption, causing a compensatory increase in the reabsorption of monovalent ions in the proximal tubule. This process can result in lithium accumulation and severe toxicity in patients receiving lithium therapy. Potassium sparing diuretics combined with potassium supplements and/or angiotensin converting enzyme (ACE) inhibitors cause hyperkalaemia.

NON-DOSE RELATED (IDIOSYNCRATIC, TYPE B) ADVERSE REACTIONS

Hypersensitivity reactions to drugs (drug allergy) involve immunological reactions. Large molecules, e.g. vaccines, insulin, dextrans, can themselves be immunogenic but most drugs are small molecules and are not antigenic on their own. In some patients (we do not know which) they, or a metabolite, act as a hapten and combine with tissue proteins, forming an antigenic conjugate. The antigens induce the synthesis of antibodies and subsequent exposure to the drug triggers an immunological reaction (e.g. rash, anaphylaxis). Although drug allergy is unpredictable, it is more likely to occur in patients with a history of atopic disease (hay fever, asthma, eczema).

Anaphylaxis is a **type I reaction** in which the drug (⬤) interacts with IgE fixed to mast cells (MC) and basophils, triggering the release of histamine and other mediators (Chapter 11). Drugs likely to cause this life-threatening reaction (top right) include penicillin, which is responsible for 75% of all anaphylactic deaths. Some drugs (e.g. some contrast media) can produce an anaphylaxis-like (anaphylactoid) reaction on first exposure.

Blood dyscrasias. Allergic reactions to drugs that cause blood dyscrasias (bottom left) involve **type II cytotoxic** reactions. Circulating antibody of the IgM or IgG type interacts with a drug (hapten) combined with the blood cell membrane to form an antigenic complex (⊶). Complement (Ⓒ) is activated, causing cell lysis. Some drugs predictably cause blood dyscrasias. For example, most cytotoxic anti-cancer agents (Chapter 43) inhibit cell division in the bone marrow, and patients with glucose-6-phosphate dehydrogenase deficiency have a high risk of haemolytic anaemia if given primaquine (Chapter 42).

Serum sickness is a **type III reaction** triggered by some drugs (bottom right), where antibody (IgG) combines with the haptenprotein antigen complex in the circulation. The resulting complex, instead of being removed normally by phagocytic cells, remains in the tissues or circulation. Phagocytic cells and complement (Ⓒ) are activated, causing inflammation and damage to the capillary endothelium. This is especially serious when the complexes are stuck to walls of vital blood vessels (e.g. renal glomeruli). The symptoms include fever, arthritis, urticaria and lymphadenopathy.

Rashes. Drugs (top left) cause a wide variety of rashes, some of which are life-threatening but fortunately rare, e.g. toxic epidermal necrolysis (35% mortality). **Type IV cell-mediated** reactions are involved in which T-lymphocytes (Ⓣ) are sensitized by a hapten–protein complex. When the lymphocytes come into contact with the antigen presenting cell (APC), an inflammatory response is produced. If the antigen (⬤) enters through the skin (e.g. antibiotic cream), contact sensitivity may cause an eczematous rash with oedema at the application site.

TERATOGENESIS

Teratogenesis is the occurrence of fetal developmental abnormalities caused by drugs taken during the first trimester of pregnancy. Most drugs cross the placental barrier to some extent and, if possible, drugs should be avoided during pregnancy. Known teratogens include alcohol (fetal alcohol syndrome), anticancer drugs, warfarin (multiple congential defects), valproate, carbamazepine (neural tube defects) and other anticonvulsants, and tetracyclines (inhibition of bone growth).

CARCINOGENESIS

Drug-induced tumours are probably very rare because the pharmaceutical industry makes great efforts to avoid marketing carcinogenic agents. The mechanisms involved in chemical carcinogenesis are usually unknown but immunosuppression (e.g. azathioprine with prednisolone) is associated with a greatly increased risk of lymphomas. Alkylating agents (e.g. cyclophosphamide) are thought to exhibit 'gene toxicity' and may cause non-lymphocytic leukaemias.

Index